'An overwhelming number of persons suffer from mental health problems across their life span. In this important book, the authors describe the critical issues in the psychiatric care of individuals with autism. Written by a father (who is an experienced psychologist), and his daughter (who has suffered from psychiatric disorders), it gives a detailed account of the difficulties faced by persons with autism and related disorders, especially as they transition into adulthood, and sheds light on the challenges faced both by patients and staff. I enjoyed reading the book and recommend it both to parents and caregivers of persons with autism and other developmental disabilities.'

Mohammad Ghaziuddin MD, Professor of Psychiatry,
University of Michigan, Ann Arbor, USA

of related interest

No Fighting, No Biting, No Screaming
How to Make Behaving Positively Possible for People
with Autism and Other Developmental Disabilities
Bo Hejlskov Elvén
ISBN 978 1 84905 126 2
eISBN 978 0 85700 322 5

Sulky, Rowdy, Rude?
Why kids really act out and what to do about it
Bo Hejlskov Elvén and Tina Wiman
ISBN 978 1 78592 213 8
eISBN 978 1 78450 492 2

Confused, Angry, Anxious?
Why working with older people in care really can
be difficult, and what to do about it
Bo Hejlskov Elvén, Charlotte Agger, and Iben Ljungmann
ISBN 978 1 78592 215 2
eISBN 978 1 78450 494 6

Disruptive, Stubborn, Out of Control?
Why kids get confrontational in the
classroom and what to do about it
Bo Hejlskov Elvén
ISBN 978 1 78592 212 1
eISBN 978 1 78450 490 8

Frightened, Disturbed, Dangerous?

Why working with patients in psychiatric care can be really difficult, and what to do about it

Bo Hejlskov Elvén and Sophie Abild McFarlane

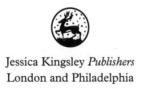

Jessica Kingsley *Publishers*
London and Philadelphia

First published in 2017
by Jessica Kingsley Publishers
73 Collier Street
London N1 9BE, UK
and
400 Market Street, Suite 400
Philadelphia, PA 19106, USA

www.jkp.com

Library of Congress Cataloging in Publication Data
A CIP catalog record for this book is available from the Library of Congress.

British Library Cataloguing in Publication Data
A CIP catalogue record for this book is available from the British Library.

ISBN: 978 1 78592 214 5
eISBN: 978 1 78450 493 9

Printed and bound in Great Britain

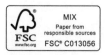

MIX
Paper from
responsible sources
FSC
www.fsc.org   FSC® C013056

Contents

Introduction

My daughter and I have written this book together. I am a psychologist and have worked for many years as a tutor and educator in schools, in disability care and in psychiatry. My daughter has been a patient in psychiatric care for 10 years, starting at 17 years of age. With this book we hope to be able to describe behaviour that challenges in psychiatric care from the perspective of both patient and staff. We have experienced psychiatry from different directions and have been able to bring together our different pictures not least because we are father and daughter.

I have worked primarily with people with disabilities, conducting investigations and training, and first encountered inpatient psychiatry as the relative of a patient. It has not always been a pleasant experience to observe my daughter Sophie's journey from the sidelines, but it has left me all the more convinced that we need to further develop the methods used in psychiatry. Since then, I have worked in psychiatry with this purpose: we need to get better at taking care of those who need it most.

When I tutor and train staff in inpatient psychiatry, I often hear a host of different stories from the staff. Many of these stories feature patients shouting, threatening, fighting or hurting themselves. But I also hear about use of methods such as sending patients to their rooms, about isolation, as-needed medication and mechanical restraint. The focus is often on what the patient should do and what the staff are doing to keep the patients calm.

Staff in psychiatry also describe the feeling of powerlessness they experience when patients act out. Psychiatric patients, in their turn, talk about staff who raise their voices, about tough demands to stay calm and about the frustration they feel over not being able to decide over themselves – and about their powerlessness. Over the years it has become my habit when working with psychiatric institutions to look specifically for this powerlessness. The reason is that the feeling of powerlessness is the most destructive emotion there is, regardless of whether we are staff, patients or relatives.

From the patient's perspective, it is easy to understand that this powerlessness is devastating. You can't influence your own life situation, you feel at the mercy of both staff and illness, and life feels like floating with the current down a river. As a patient in psychiatry, the river is wild, throwing you back and forth against the rocks and sometimes under the water. For the staff, the sense of powerlessness is just as devastating. Helpless staff are often confrontational and demanding towards patients. We who are staff can be cynical and resigned, and can at times become so helpless that we try to avoid the very patients for whom we are assigned to care.

The powerlessness in the system – the shared powerlessness experienced by both staff and patients – is probably the worst. Instead of dealing with this powerlessness together, staff and patients become increasingly opposed to each other. There is often an atmosphere of mutual distrust. In these situations, both patients and staff resort to behaviours and methods that don't have the desired effect. This is the ultimate consequence of powerlessness.

PSYCHIATRY'S MOST IMPORTANT TASK

Psychiatry's task is to diagnose and treat. Behaviour that challenges causes a disruption and should therefore be handled simply and smoothly so that psychiatry can concentrate on its task. Psychiatry's task is not to instruct or treat patients in such a way that they learn to behave properly. The task consists of managing and preventing negative behaviours that can delay the patient's development towards a functioning life – and preferably with methods that don't take too much space, time and energy. So it is not the patient's task to behave; instead, it is psychiatry's task to create contexts that *help* the patient to behave so that psychiatry can fulfil its task of treatment.

THE PURPOSE OF THIS BOOK

The book you are holding is an attempt to address the unfortunate lack of knowledge that exists in psychiatry about how to effectively and professionally – and based on scientific research – handle behaviour that challenges. By considering approaches and methods, it is possible to make a marked difference in everyday life in psychiatric wards as well as in outpatient care and social psychiatry.

This book is about how we as staff can behave towards patients so that they develop towards a functioning life, with self-determination and the possibility to take responsibility for their actions. It is directed primarily towards staff in inpatient facilities and in social psychiatry, but staff in outpatient care may also benefit from the methods and view of humanity presented in the book. The focus of the book is the management of behaviour that challenges, not treatment, and will therefore probably be most useful to those working with patients on a broader scale than just therapy.

No diagnoses are named in the book. This is intentional. Diagnoses are important for treatment and prognoses, but at the moment when someone is fighting or throwing furniture around, diagnoses are not important.

THE STRUCTURE OF THE BOOK

The book is divided into three parts. The first part has 11 chapters, each of which brings up and discusses one principle. A principle, in this case, is defined as a foundational statement and as something towards which one should strive. The first chapter, for example, is based on the principle 'Always identify who it is that has a problem'.

These principles are included in an approach called the low-arousal approach and they build on research into the management of behaviour that challenges. I hope that these principles will suffice to create an openness, and to get us to try thinking and acting differently. When one dares to do so, one often sees results that are both effective and good. But it requires both flexibility and openness from you as a reader.

The principles are all illustrated by means of a situation from everyday life (i.e. a case description). The situations are ones that the co-author, my daughter Sophie, has experienced as a patient in psychiatric wards and psychiatric residences. Let's allow Sophie to introduce herself:

> The picture of mutual powerlessness, of violence and conflict, that is described above is something that I,

Sophie, have experienced first-hand. I have been a patient in psychiatry's inpatient and outpatient care, in social psychiatry and in psychiatric residences during the more than 10 years that have passed since I was 17 years old. My contribution to this book is the case descriptions with which the chapters begin and on which they are built. They are situations that I or my fellow patients have experienced as inpatients or in psychiatric residences. All the situations are, of course, anonymised, except for the fact that you now know I was there. Today I have a good life and live with my fiancé in a small townhouse, and I manage with outpatient care. So luckily I no longer experience situations like those described in this book. While I am in a good situation, I hope to be able to contribute to the development of treatment methods within psychiatry.

The behaviour of the staff in some of the cases described may appear both indefensible and unethical. In this book, I don't intend to point out what the staff did wrong. I am convinced that you as a reader can determine that yourself. Most of the situations are situations that go wrong because the methods that are used are not good. One of the purposes of the book is to help staff find better work methods, so that treatment becomes safer for both patient and staff, gives a better chance of success and also gets better from an ethical point of view. To achieve this purpose, we as staff sometimes need to be confronted by ourselves and our methods.

The second part of the book provides more examples of situations from Sophie's life, where we consider the situations in the light of the principles dealt with in the first part. By reviewing the situations, we can understand what is happening and formulate a possible strategy for how one could handle the situation in a different way.

This book is based on research into how people behave and what works and doesn't work in healthcare, care of people with disabilities and pedagogy. Except in a few cases, I have not included references in the text since I feel that this makes it harder to read, but if you want to go to the sources, in Part 3, at the end of the book is an extended bibliography (see Further Reading) which describes, chapter by chapter, the basis for the text. There is also study material that can be used as a basis for discussion during staff meetings.

Part 1

Principles

Part 1 consists of a number of principles for behaviour management in the low-arousal tradition. Every chapter starts with a case illustrating the principle of the chapter.

1

Always Identify Who It Is That Has a Problem

ASHLEY

Ashley is voluntarily committed to a ward. Sometimes she has difficulty falling asleep at night and lies in bed, twisting and turning. And so, during her most recent conversation with the ward doctor, Ashley asked for some sleeping pills. The doctor advised against her taking more medicine but thought she should drink a hot cup of tea before going to bed. That would most likely help her relax and get to sleep for the night.

In this ward, patients are not allowed to go to bed until after the evening medicines have been distributed at 10 p.m. By that time, however, the patients' tea trolley has long since been removed.

A couple of days after speaking with her doctor, Ashley decides to try his advice. She goes to the staffroom to ask for some tea, since the tea trolley has already been taken away.

Maybe the staff can make an exception for her? But the staff in the kitchen don't want to give Ashley any tea. Ashley asks: 'But look, you have tea there. Can't you just give me a cup of that?' No, the staff don't want to do that.

There are rules for when tea should be served to patients, and how would it be if everyone wanted tea at night?

Ashley gets stressed, starts crying and sits down on the floor in the corridor. A healthcare assistant, Deacon, comes out of the staffroom, takes her by the arm and lifts her up to a standing position, saying: 'You go off to your room now and go to sleep.' Ashley tries to get free by flinging out her arms, which has the result that she catches Deacon in the stomach and he falls over. Deacon presses the alarm button. When a member of staff sounds the alarm at night, healthcare assistants respond from two different wards. A total of six healthcare assistants wrestle Ashley to the floor, hold her down and give her an injection. Then she is put in her bed and taken away to a locked ward. It takes two weeks before she is back in the open ward.

WHO SOLVES ASHLEY'S PROBLEM?

The principle 'Always identify who it is that has a problem' is important. In the example above, Ashley is prescribed by the doctor to drink tea in order to fall asleep more easily. When she tries to do this, she runs into resistance that she experiences as frustrating and possibly insulting. Her reaction is to cry in the corridor, and then to fling out her arms to get free of the healthcare assistant who is trying to help her. The reaction to this is massive, and the outcome is two weeks in a locked ward.

For the reader this doesn't seem like a reasonable solution. But from the staff's perspective, Ashley is a problem. She isn't following the framework of rules that the staff must follow. She cries and doesn't want to go to bed, and she causes one of the workers to risk hurting himself when he falls.

Ashley has very little freedom of action, but she feels she has the right to react to what she perceives as injustice, and the means she has at her disposal are crying or trying to get free. This means that there isn't really any incentive for Ashley to change behaviour. She is handling a difficult situation in the only ways available to her.

If the staff start from the assumption that it is Ashley who has a behaviour problem, things will get difficult. In that case they will want Ashley to change her behaviour. But she doesn't think that her behaviour is a problem and is unable to see how she could come up with a different solution. It is therefore necessary for the staff to determine how to make sure this doesn't happen again. The staff's incentive to change the situation must be greater than Ashley's incentive. They are professionals. Ashley is a patient with documented difficulties in managing in life and everyday routine. To forcefully drag Ashley away to a locked ward is not reasonable, and not a good solution. Reasons for involuntary care should have to do with the patient being a danger to himself or to others. And the danger must be significant. Here it is not.

WHY IT'S NOT UP TO THE PATIENT TO SOLVE PSYCHIATRY'S PROBLEMS

This book is about how we can get to grips with problems that we may encounter as staff in psychiatry and social psychiatry. But it is very important, right from the start, to point out that the focus is on differentiating between what is the staff's problem and what is the patient's problem. The reason for this is that the book deals primarily with methods the staff can use to solve problems that arise in everyday work, so that the work runs more smoothly and doesn't drain their own energy.

Patients often try to solve their problems with the means they have at hand. But as mentioned earlier, they are in psychiatric care because they have trouble managing their daily routine, their feelings and their life. Therefore, the staff have a greater responsibility than the patients. We are professionals; the patients are not. Therefore, it is we who bear the responsibility. Only by taking responsibility can we solve the problems we encounter.

NICOLE
Nicole is being moved from psychiatric emergency to the ward. During the move she has the hood of her light jacket up in order to screen off impressions. The staff ask her to take off her jacket. Nicole doesn't want to do so. The staff tell her a few more times, and when Nicole persists in not removing her jacket, they pull down her hood. Nicole waits for a while and then pulls it up again.

In Nicole's case, too, there is a reason for her behaviour. She is not feeling well and needs to screen herself off. The staff don't understand this and pull down her hood. But Nicole is a woman of resource; she is patient and pulls the hood back up after a while. It is clear that the staff have a problem with Nicole having her hood up. Nicole's problem is that there's too much going on around her and that the staff are taking off her hood. This means that they have two different problems and therefore two different solutions. To expect Nicole to try to understand and solve the staff's problem is probably not realistic.

Summary

It's an everyday occurrence in psychiatry and social psychiatry that we handle behaviour that challenges as if it is the patient who has a problem, whereas in actual fact it is the staff who think there is a problem. A patient who doesn't see or think that there is a problem seldom feels motivated to change his behaviour. It is therefore the professional staff's responsibility to change the situation so that behaviour that challenges doesn't occur.

2

People Behave Well
If They Can

ZOE

The staff at the psychiatric residence have invited everyone to have dinner together at 6 p.m., but they haven't brought enough food. Zoe is clearly stressed by the situation. She's not very comfortable in large groups and likes to eat alone. And the time has reached 6:15 p.m. before the food is on the table.

Zoe wanders back and forth in the room and tries to talk to the staff about what they are going to eat. The staff eventually get tired of this and ask her to take her portion and go to her room. In the rush Zoe takes a little more food than she usually eats. The staff ask her to put some salad back, which makes her irritated, and she starts to argue back. In the end the staff try to lead her out of the room. Zoe gets angry, shouts and screams, throws the food on the floor and then goes out to have a smoke in the yard.

ABILITIES, DEMANDS AND EXPECTATIONS

The principle 'People behave well if they can' was formulated by psychologist Ross W. Greene. The principle is actually very simple. If a person behaves well, it is because he is *able* to do so. If a person does not behave well, it is because he *cannot* do so – and then those around him need to begin to think about whether they are placing too high demands on the person's abilities.

In Zoe's case in the example above, there are various demands and expectations of necessary abilities in the different stages of the event described. One such ability might be to manage to do something out of the ordinary.

On normal days Zoe makes her own food together with her support staff and eats by herself. Suddenly something happens that is out of the ordinary: she is going to eat with the other residents – and be nice even. The very thought makes her feel stressed. And when the food takes time in appearing, Zoe's restlessness increases. The ability to wait involves endurance, and Zoe's endurance is quite limited. She gets more and more impatient.

Add to this the demand that Zoe should be able to adapt when the staff notice that the situation is not ideal. They quickly change plans. This can be a good thing in itself, especially if it is done because they see that Zoe is getting stressed – but also hard to take. For many patients, stressful situations imply reduced flexibility. They have difficulty in adapting quickly.

Zoe does her best. She starts to take food. Because of her level of stress, she doesn't manage to suit the amount of food to the situation, only to her hunger. When the staff then ask her to put some food back, it's just too much. She feels shame because she took too much, frustration because she's not allowed to eat enough to get full, anger because the staff made her feel embarrassed and childish, and maybe sudden sadness at the fact that she lives in a residence and can't escape this type of situation. She can't navigate any longer and challenges authority; she argues back.

The staff don't want their authority challenged. They increase their level of intervention by trying to lead her out. This increases Zoe's sense of powerlessness, so she starts shouting and screaming. Luckily, the staff let go. Here the situation could have escalated further and ended in physical restraint and violence. Zoe throws the food down and then on her own initiative goes out into the yard to calm down.

In summary, Zoe has difficulties in readjusting, in being part of a larger context, in structuring and calculating quantity, in calculating the consequences of her behaviour and in regulating her affect. But she does her best throughout the situation. Her best just isn't good enough.

Zoe is by no means an unusual patient in psychiatry. Most psychiatric patients have problems in getting their everyday life to hang together. The difficulties they experience vary, but in this situation the demands and expectations on Zoe's abilities were too much for her.

CHARACTERISTICS AND NORMAL DISTRIBUTION

Human characteristics are often normally distributed in the population. This applies to characteristics such as height, weight, intelligence, attentiveness, ability to structure, learning ability, ability to wait, social abilities and a host of other things. Normal distribution is often illustrated as in Figure 2.1.

Figure 2.1 should be understood as a group of people placed on a line based on a characteristic such as height: short people to the left and tall people to the right. In the middle are those of average height, which means most people, so the line forms a hump here. This illustrates that most people's characteristics lie around the average. The further we move from the average, regardless of direction, the fewer people we will encounter. This is easy to understand when it comes to height, but exactly the same thing applies to the abilities that the food situation demanded in Zoe's case. If one falls way below the average in any of these abilities, for example affect regulation, the risk (or chance) increases that one will receive a diagnosis.

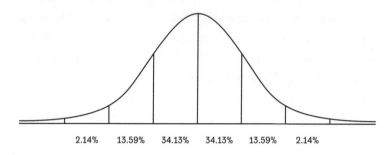

2.14%   13.59%   34.13%   34.13%   13.59%   2.14%

Figure 2.1 The normal distribution curve

But there is a gradual transition between diagnosis and normal. This means that in everyday life in psychiatry, and in psychiatric residences such as in Zoe's case, there will be people who manage a deviation from everyday routine very well, many who manage well, a few who manage more or less, and a couple who have major problems when the routine is replaced by new demands. The shape of the day also plays a role: most patients (just like everyone else) manage situations better when they feel good themselves.

PEOPLE'S RESOURCES VARY

A central theme throughout this book is that people's resources and abilities vary. In discussing behaviour that challenges I am speaking about those who have the resources to live up to the demands we place on them and those who do not.

There can be many reasons for not being able to live up to demands and expectations; it may be stress – for example, problematic relationships or insecurity in one's daily life. But in this book I am not discussing patients' will to behave or their intentions. The most important reason for this is that research has shown that if we work on the basis of Greene's principle 'People behave well if they can', then we become more effective in our work. It often goes a long way in helping us solve the situations that arise in our daily work.

PART OF EVERYDAY LIFE

There will always be situations that don't go as planned or as we want them to do. Sometimes I am surprised by the way in which staff talk about behaviour that challenges as if it were a deviation from the norm. It isn't. It's part of everyday life. But every time we have a situation that goes badly, we should sit down and think about what went wrong. In the various phases of the situation's development we will see exactly where we were making demands that were too high – if we search. But if we only try to see what the patient *should* have done – instead of what he did – then we will have problems next time we end up in a similar situation. We only see that the situation didn't turn out well – we don't see a solution.

So we must examine our own behaviour and our own expectations of the patient's abilities in order to then be able to compare them with the patient's real abilities. Then it won't be so hard to see where the problems lie. If the patient didn't behave well, then we will find some area in which we ourselves didn't succeed. That's how it is. It may be hard to accept, but that's how it is.

It requires a lot of the staff in such situations to see their own role in the patient's behaviour, but this is absolutely essential if the situation is not to be repeated. All behaviour occurs as an interplay with the environment – either a direct interplay with us or an interplay with the environment we control.

DEMANDS THAT ARE TOO HIGH

Conflicts arise because the situation places demands that are too high on the patient's abilities. Are we perhaps asking too much of the ability to create structure or to control impulses, or of the patient's social skills?

If one has been through a time-consuming conflict, one should immediately create a plan to prevent this type of conflict from happening again. What should the everyday routine look like in order to reduce the risk of conflict? Should all patients be in communal areas at the same time? Should there be more staff available at certain times? Should there be more planned activities for some of the patients?

We need to evaluate whether we have too high expectations of the following abilities from our patients:

- *Ability to calculate cause and effect in complex settings*
  This is required in order to calculate the consequences of our own actions, but also in order to create for ourselves a picture of what is going to happen overall. Patients who struggle with this need much more structure and predictability than others.

- *Ability to structure, plan and carry out activities*
  Many patients are unable to create an overview of a morning and plan what they will do, and they don't know how much they still have left of a current activity.

- *Ability to remember while thinking*
  This ability is usually called working memory. Some patients cannot both remember and process the information they have in their heads at the same time. In such cases when you can't use spoken instructions, you may have to write or draw what they are to do.

- *Ability to restrain impulses*
  Many patients react immediately to whatever is happening and simply can't resist impulses when they come. We must therefore think about the impulses we are creating through our rules and the way we act towards people. Rules that are about something you mustn't do create the impulse to do that thing.

- *Endurance*
  Some patients find it much harder to wait than others. The same patients often have difficulty in performing activities that require long periods of concentration.

- *Flexibility or the ability to readjust quickly*
  Most people prefer things to be the same way as usual, and some have great difficulty in handling change – even when the change is inevitable and the staff think they are just being silly.

- *Social skills, such as calculating how other people will think, feel and act*
  Some patients have tremendous difficulty in seeing their own role in things that go wrong and in understanding how their behaviour is perceived by others. These people often find it difficult to evaluate other people's intentions.

- *Sensitivity to stress*
  The amount of stress we can take varies. Patients in inpatient care are usually overly stressed. In open care and social psychiatry there may be stress in other parts of life that make it difficult for patients to cooperate in matters related to their care.

- *Ability to say yes*
  It sounds strange, but some people say yes to most things in life, and some say no. This is a personality trait that is not easily changed, but it can be compensated for. If a patient has difficulty in saying yes, we must increase their sense of participation, for example by providing more options from which to choose.

- *Ability to calm down and stay calm*
  We call this the ability to regulate affect. This ability varies from person to person and increases with age. But it is an ability, not a matter of will. No one wants to lose control over their feelings.

SHOWING CONSIDERATION WHERE NEEDED

Greene's work involves helping people to develop abilities where we make demands that are too high. This book does not do that. This book is about how to make everyday life simple and good for people who spend most of their time as psychiatric patients. We do this not by spending lots of time getting patients motivated to accept treatment, but rather by showing the consideration needed for all patients to be able to cooperate with us.

We don't know if Greene's principle 'People behave well if they can' is true, but we do know that it is effective. That's enough for me. If we think in this way, conflicts are reduced, patients are happy and develop, and the staff's experience of success increases.

Summary

People behave well if they can. If a patient is not behaving well, we most likely have too high demands and expectations of the patient's abilities. To change this, we can examine the expectations we have in situations that go wrong and then adjust them so that they fit better with what the patient can be expected to manage.

3

People Do What Makes Sense

CONNOR

Connor has been feeling unwell for some time. This morning his mother came by and saw the state he was in. Connor was lying in bed and his home was a mess. He seemed tired and sad. His mother tried talking with him and then they took a taxi to the psychiatric emergency ward, where he was admitted. But the ward itself was full, so Connor had to lie in the corridor.

It's an old hospital with a long corridor. All sounds in the corridor can be heard for a long way. Connor gets stressed by being there. What he really wants is peace and quiet, but staff are running back and forth in the corridor all the time. Suddenly another patient gets violent in the waiting room. The patient shouts and flails at those around him. The staff press the alarm and ten healthcare assistants come running. They wrestle down the patient and drag him to the restraining room, right past Connor's bed.

After a while, Connor starts to sing. It sounds wonderful to sing in the corridor: there are good acoustics and lots of echoes. And it shuts out all the other sounds. A patient walking past tells him it sounds damn awful and calls him a 'bloody loudmouth'. Connor starts to cry. He cries louder and louder. Other patients start getting restless because of his crying and, after a while, a member of staff comes and asks him how he is feeling.

ACTIONS THAT MAKE SENSE

Most of us try to do what makes the most sense in the situation in which we happen to be. There are many examples of this. Regardless of the speed limit shown on the traffic sign, for example, we tend to drive more slowly on narrow roads than on broader ones – and even slower if the road has many curves. Slowing down when the road gets narrower is the most logical thing to do. In the same way, it is a completely logical and understandable action for a preschool child to jump into an inviting puddle. To choose anything else requires an active impulse control. What makes sense, then, is not so much about what you understand, but about what you do when you're not really thinking about it – just like Connor singing when the acoustics are good.

I have often found that staff think you can change a patient's behaviour by talking to him or her. I don't think so. 'Surely you can understand...' is not the way to success when the patient can't calculate cause and effect in complex situations. For many psychiatric patients this ability is missing all the time, and all of us lose it when we are stressed. And being stressed is probably the best common description of patients in psychiatry.

RULES THAT DON'T MAKE SENSE

One of the most common behaviour problems is that patients don't follow the rules. When I talk about this with staff, most of them seem to think that of course you have to follow the rules. And if a problem arises, it is not unusual that the first action taken is to impose a new rule. I usually ask staff in such situations whether they follow all of society's rules. It always turns out that they do not. People follow the rules that make sense and that seem meaningful to them. We have trouble following rules that don't make sense.

A good example of a rule that doesn't make sense to many is that one should not wear a hat or cap indoors. This is a fully understandable rule for people born before, say, 1975. The reason may be that an important factor in what makes sense is habit. If one was raised when it was not the done thing to wear a hat or cap indoors, then it makes sense. But for people born after 1975 it isn't quite so obvious – maybe because for people born before 1975, a cap or hat is a practical item of clothing, with a focus on staying warm, whereas for people born after 1975 it has to do with appearance and identity. As a result, suddenly we have staff who wear a cap or hat indoors and rules have had to be changed in many places.

The important thing if patients don't obey a rule like this, however, is that it doesn't make sense to remove one's hat when going inside if the hat is an expression of your identity. If we require patients to be hat- or cap-free indoors, then we will have to remind and nag every day. And that has its price. Patients will think that staff who are always nagging about hats are idiots. This ruins the treatment alliance – that is, the trust and confidence that the patient must feel for the staff in order to benefit from treatment. I would go so far as to say that the rule about not having a cap or hat on indoors contributes to fewer patients eventually succeeding in leading a functioning life. This doesn't affect everyone, but it has great importance in the group of patients where head covering is an important part of their identity.

SHORTCUTS TO SENSE

If one chooses to work with the concept of making sense as a principle, then there are some shortcuts available. It is often good to begin with the physical framework. Building away behaviour that challenges is often the cheapest option. Calm colours, rooms with quiet acoustics and technology that makes doors close quietly instead of with a bang create a restful environment. A chaotic environment often leads to a more chaotic daily life. This may seem like a minor detail, but in my experience it is one of the most important and easiest things we can do.

Another shortcut is to create sense through predictability. Many patients have no problem getting calmly through the day if they have an overview of what they are going to do and for how long (just like most other people, including those who aren't patients). Creating a plan for the day and making it visible to the patients considerably reduces behaviour that challenges.

One must also remember to cross out activities that are completed, to improve the overview. A few patients may need a plan for the day on their own piece of paper, an investment which I have seen the value of time and time again. Some patients may also need more concrete details than others in order to increase meaningfulness. Once again: patients' resources differ, and behaviour that challenges arises when we expect patients to have abilities that they don't have.

The same thing applies to spare time. An activity that makes sense is better for some patients than just taking it easy – not least if the patient has a tendency to engage in self-harming behaviour. Some patients have found a solution in applying themselves to a recurring activity, such as playing cards.

Summary

People always do the thing that makes the most sense in the situation. It is therefore easier to understand behaviour that challenges by looking at how the behaviour makes sense to the patient. If we want to change the situation, we can create prerequisites for how the patient is expected to act – by making the desired behaviour the one that makes the most sense in the situation.

4

The One Who Takes Responsibility Can Make a Difference

PAIGE

Paige is in hospital and has had her medication changed. She's 19 years old. The new medicine causes her to lactate, which, in her psychosis, she finds terrifying. So she asks to speak to the doctor about it. The ward staff promise to arrange a meeting with the doctor.

On day two the doctor doesn't come. Neither does the doctor come on day three. On the morning of day four the nurse comes into Paige's room with the morning medication. Paige refuses to take it. She says: 'You promised that I would get to talk to the doctor about the milk in my breasts, but nothing's happening. I don't want to take this disgusting medicine. I want to talk to the doctor.' The nurse says: 'If you won't even take your medicine, then why are you here?' Paige bangs her head hard against the wall three times and starts to bleed. The nurse leaves the room but sends a nursing aide to dress Paige's wounds.

An hour later, Paige goes to see the head nurse and demands to see the doctor at once. She is told to calm down, which makes her start shouting really loudly, throw a chair and scream. She is then mechanically restrained for an hour until she has calmed down again.

Later in the day, Paige is called into the head nurse's office and told that she can't go around blackmailing the staff by hurting herself or throwing furniture around. She just has to wait until the doctor has time to talk to her. If this behaviour is repeated, Paige is told, then she will be moved to a locked ward.

WHO IS RESPONSIBLE?

The principle 'The one who takes responsibility can make a difference' was formulated by psychologist Bernhard Weiner. It spread very widely in occupational psychology with concepts such as 'influencing one's own work environment' – something that proved able to reduce sick leave and improve well-being at workplaces. In the context of care, psychologist Dave Dagnan has taken Weiner's ideas the furthest. He has studied how staff perceive patients' behaviour, and their views on the patient's ability to control his own behaviour, matter a great deal with regard to how effective the treatment proves to be.

In the example with Paige above, it gets very difficult if the staff think that a conversation in the office with Paige about her behaviour will prevent the same thing from happening again – because this means that Paige is the one who must make sure that it doesn't happen again. Unfortunately, it also means that if it does happen again, then the staff are at a total loss as to what to do. If their way of dealing with an event is to place the responsibility on the patient, then the staff are left powerless and have no possibility of resolving the situation. Powerless staff are a big problem and not the way to go if one wants to reduce behaviour that challenges.

In his research, Dave Dagnan has examined what happens when staff believe that the patient is violent or self-harming on purpose, as compared with when they believe that he is doing his best but not succeeding. The results are astonishing. Staff who think that Paige is responsible for her own behaviour in a situation like this will, first of all, experience many similar situations. They will also experience the powerlessness that comes from being unable to influence someone's behaviour. This means that they will go to work every day in fear and trepidation of how badly things will go. It can get so bad that it will depend on Paige whether or not the staff have a good day. For things to be this way will lead to increased absence due to illness and greater turnover of staff. This in turn will have negative effects on the quality of treatment for all the patients.

On the other hand, if they decide that Paige did her best, but that she found it difficult having milk running from her breasts, then suddenly they have the possibility to make changes that may prevent the same thing from happening again. Above all, they have the possibility of influencing their situation and, in the long run, their work. This will lead to less absence due to illness, less staff turnover, and better development and treatment effects for patients.

PUNISHMENT AND CONSEQUENCES

It is in situations such as Paige's situation that one most often finds staff who feel provoked. They may say: 'Should the patient really be allowed to act and talk like that? Shouldn't there be consequences?' This is an interesting argument. First, there is probably no one who thinks it is OK for Paige to hurt herself or to fight – least of all Paige. But in a difficult situation she is doing her best, and it doesn't turn out very well. The situation is as it is. This we have to relate to. So the question is what can help reduce the risk of it happening again. That's where consequences come in. Most people think that if you experience a negative consequence after a certain behaviour, then the behaviour will diminish – because that's how we think it is for *us*.

The difference between punishment and functioning consequences has been discussed by psychologists, sociologists and pedagogues for many years. If one looks at the available research, there is really only one factor that is interesting: If the person feels that he is being punished, then in the long term the problem behaviour increases. So it is not a matter of what actually happens but how it is perceived by the patient. The consequences that we remember and that we think helped us are not those we experienced as punishment.

Punishment is something about which we know much more. For example, we know that:

- *Punishment most often makes you feel unfairly treated.* For staff this shouldn't come as a surprise. Patients often say: 'What? It wasn't just me!' when we intervene and punish. To feel unfairly treated by staff means that the relationship between staff and patients takes a knock. This relationship, or alliance, is central to treatment.

- *Punishment increases the very behaviour we are punishing.* This is true both on the community and the individual level. It is the reason why first-time offenders often receive conditional sentences. An unconditional sentence results in a 150% higher recurrence rate compared with a conditional sentence.

- *Punishment can legitimise behaviour that challenges.*
  Research by the American economists Gneezy and Rustichini has shown that you can double the number of children still at preschool at closing time if you institute fines for picking up your children late. The reason is that the punishment removes the bad conscience. If I am willing to pay the price, then I don't need to have a bad conscience. This effect goes both ways.

- *We have differing tendencies to punish.*
  This effect we can call the de Quervain effect after the Swiss neurophysiologist Dominique de Quervain. Together with some colleagues (de Quervain *et al.* 2004), she studied two things: partly whether there are differences in people who punish, and partly why we do it. They came up with the following answer: Different people have different tendencies to punish. One can predict who will be the most likely to punish by measuring brain activity in an area of the brain called the dorsal striatum, often referred to as the brain's reward centre. The greater the activity, the greater the tendency to punish. But the most interesting thing was that everyone received a personal sense of reward when they punished someone else. It simply felt good! Even if one actually lost something by punishing someone, one still received a feeling of competence and justice. There has been speculation as to why this is so. One of those with a theory is evolution psychologist Robert Boyd. He thinks that, in prehistoric times, those who got rid of people who were spoiling things for the flock or the village by throwing them out before they could do too much harm survived better than those who did not. That is why we have developed this reward effect

when we punish others. In psychiatry, however, we are meant to care for those who are constantly being thrown out of various situations. This means that we can't resort to an evolutionary mechanism that focuses on group survival every time a patient swears at a member of staff.

The question is not whether the patient should be allowed to say or do the things he does. The question is really about how to make sure he doesn't do it again. And that brings us back to the title of the previous chapter: 'People Behave Well If They Can'. What was it in the situation that made it unmanageable for Paige? How can we create different conditions so that things go better next time?

HITTING THE SKILL CEILING

Staff are quite good at taking responsibility when they have a good method. If we know what to do and what works, then we will do it willingly. But sometimes we end up in situations where we don't have a functioning method. We lack the necessary skills. This we can call 'hitting the skill ceiling'. At this point we have a tendency to immediately pass the responsibility to someone else. It may be to lay the responsibility on the patient by punishing him (with an argument such as: then maybe he'll learn; he must take responsibility) or by yelling, shouting and scolding. Sometimes I think that staff members think: *He has to behave, and if he doesn't understand that, I'll have to say it again, but louder so that he understands.*

Another example can be to place the responsibility on one's boss or on the politicians. We can do this by saying: 'This patient's behaviour is so bad that he shouldn't be here with us. He should be in a locked forensic psychiatry ward.' Some patients need more support than can be provided in social psychiatry or in supported living residences. But it is fairer to say that we are unable to adjust our efforts to the patient's needs than to say that he doesn't belong in our care. In most cases it is more about our unwillingness or inability to make the adjustments that are needed for the patient to be able to manage in our care. We can also try to avoid responsibility by demanding that the patient behave himself, threaten with compelling measures or hold conversations about how the patient should be acting. If our only intervention is to talk to the patient about what he should be doing, then it is actually most likely because we don't know what *we* should do.

If we are to succeed in our care assignment, then we simply must adjust our method. To talk about what the patient should know or should do will not help us better fulfil our assignment, but may rather lead us to stop exerting ourselves. Then we are seriously failing our patient. If the patient's behaviour results in him being excluded from fellowship with others, this increases our responsibility and our workload. It does not reduce the requirement to succeed. If we are to succeed, therefore, we must recognise when we have reached the skill ceiling. This is perhaps one of the most important things with which we need to work.

As staff, we are professionals. We simply must make use of methods that work. So we need to know what works, and not least, evaluate whether what we are doing is having a good effect. So if we have talked with a patient about what he should do and it hasn't helped, this is not the patient's fault. The fact that talking doesn't work is, as mentioned before, probably because we have too high expectations of the patient's ability.

A principle often used is: 'The one who does the same thing ten times and expects a different result the tenth time is crazy!' One has to agree. So one method of recognising when one has reached the skill ceiling is to count. Have I tried this several times before? Did it work then? If not, why should I do it again? When we reach the skill ceiling and start placing responsibility for patients' behaviour on the patients themselves, our bosses and politicians, or other people, then we lose the possibility of influencing patients' behaviour. We will become ineffective, absence due to illness will probably increase, and the risk of suffering a breakdown will increase greatly.

Summary
By accepting responsibility, we can create possibilities for influencing our own situation. If we think that others should solve the problems we encounter, then we lose that possibility and become powerless. We must therefore avoid methods that place the responsibility anywhere but on ourselves. Therefore, we must avoid punishment, consequences and reprimands when we want to influence a patient's behaviour.

REFERENCE

de Quervain, D.J.F., Fischbacher, U., Treyer, V., Schellhammer, M. *et al.* (2004) 'The neural basis of altruistic punishment.' *Science 305*, 1254–1258.

5

Those Who Are Used to Failing Learn Nothing from Failing One More Time

RHYS

Rhys plays the guitar and he loves hard rock. It's a big part of his life and identity. He has played since he was a child, and as a teenager he played in several bands. Now as an adult he meets with a friend once or twice a month and they jam together. Rhys dresses like a hard rocker, with piercings, keychain and black clothes. His hair is long and black.

Rhys lives in a psychiatric residence and plays electric guitar in his apartment – often loudly. He often wants to play for the staff, especially for a young woman, Emma, who also likes hard rock. Emma doesn't know how to tell him, but she doesn't think he's very good. She thinks it sounds off. One day she picks up her courage and says: 'Rhys, you will probably never be a rock star. Are you sure you're good enough?'

Contrary to her fears, Rhys doesn't get at all angry or sad. He says: 'Of course I won't. It sounds like shit. But what the hell, I'm not good at anything else either.'

DO WE LEARN FROM SUCCESS OR FAILURE?

The principle 'Those who are used to failing learn nothing from failing one more time' builds on research by neuropsychologist Anna van Duivenvoorde and her colleagues in Holland. In 2008, they were able to show that children under 15 years of age didn't learn by finding out that what they had done wasn't good. In their research they used a magnetic resonance imaging camera to measure how the brain functions during various activities. The experiment was simple: Each participant was given a number of tasks to solve in approximately 15 minutes. They were not told how they should solve them. If they solved a problem well, they received praise in the form of: 'Now it was right.' When they did wrong, they were told: 'Now it was wrong.' The research group was interested in discovering whether the neurological mechanisms for learning were the same regardless of whether we learned from success or from failure.

The results were totally unexpected. When a teenager who had turned 15 years old was told 'Now it was wrong', brain activity increased in certain parts of the brain that we know have to do with learning. If the same person was told 'Now it was right', then brain activity in the same areas dropped markedly. When the same experiment was done with children under the age of 11 years, the results were the opposite. When they learned that they had done right, the activity increased; when they learned they were wrong, the activity diminished.

Van Duivenvoorde and colleagues interpreted the increase in activity as an indication of learning, which means that people over 15 years old learn by failing, while children under 11 years of age learn by succeeding. In the 11- to 15-years age group, there were variations from child to child, which the research group interpreted to mean that children develop from learning by success to learning by failure at this age.

The theory builds on the concept that we learn by deviation from the norm. Normally developed children fail all the time when they are small. With age, however, they become more skilful, and some time before the age of 15 years, most start to succeed more often than they fail.

When they are little, children are surprised when they succeed; as adults we are surprised when we fail. This is one of the reasons that many give up a sport or stop playing a musical instrument around the age of 13 to 15 years. We suddenly discover that we're not very good. Only those who are very good keep going. This also means that, as normal and well-functioning adults, we are not surprised when someone tells us that we are good at something. In the same way, children are not at all surprised when something goes wrong. They make the same mistake over and over again – and just keep going – because they are not expecting to do it right (just like Rhys in the example above).

WHY REPRIMANDS DON'T WORK

If we are to take the research by van Duivenvoorde and colleagues seriously, then we must refrain from reprimanding children under the age of 15 years. Presumably it has no effect. On the other hand, it might be a good idea to tell them what to do next time in order to succeed. And we can certainly tell them when they succeed, preferably by praising their efforts: 'You worked very well. And you succeeded too. You got it right!'

Well-functioning youths over the age of 15 years and adults can be corrected by calmly explaining what went wrong. But only if it is *unusual* for things to go wrong. For the young people who continue to fail, correction has no effect whatsoever. Only those who have started to get it right more often than wrong can benefit from correction. And this is where it suddenly becomes relevant to psychiatry. Succeeding in life is, among other things, about not ending up in institutional or social psychiatric care. Many psychiatric patients have never reached the point where they succeed more often than they fail. Some patients have started to succeed, but then reverted to failing more often again in connection with the onset of the psychiatric condition. Common to inpatients in institutions is that they, at least for the moment, fail more than they succeed. This means that most of them have actually started to expect to fail. And so they are not surprised when someone tells them that they have failed again. There are those who, even as adults, are surprised when something goes well.

HOW THE PERSON WHO IS USED TO FAILING LEARNS FROM SUCCESS

The fact that people who are used to failing don't learn from failure – but rather from success – means that the argument 'If we don't point out that the patient has done wrong, he won't learn anything' becomes meaningless. If we have a good outer framework in which we adjust ourselves to the patient's resources, then he will succeed and thereby learn something. This also means that the patient might possibly become so used to succeeding that he, in the normal way, can begin to learn from failure. The more the patient fails, the less he will learn from it, even in the long run. So the argument 'If we adjust too much then the patient won't learn anything' is also wrong. Here is a little reading comprehension exercise: people who are used to failing can only learn from failure by first succeeding a great deal.

Often when we use punishment or reprimands we try to solve an immediate problem but at the same time avoid the situation being repeated. We do that by pushing buttons on the patient. We wrongly assume that if this situation is a bad situation, the patient will avoid repeating it by changing his or her behaviour. That never works.

We have an important principle here. We cannot solve a situation here and now and at the same time prevent that it will happen again. We need to apply a model of situation management and change that reads:

1. Manage the situation without escalating the situation.

2. Evaluate. What went wrong?

3. Change what needs to be changed in order to avoid repeating the situation next time.

That way, we can both solve our immediate problem and avoid that it will happen again – but by taking responsibility instead of placing it on the patient. This means that we keep the possibility of making a difference.

Summary
Most adults learn something every time they fail. That is why most people only make the same mistake a few times. Children, however, can fail in the same way over and over again without finding it a problem. They learn by succeeding instead. Psychiatric patients have rarely managed to develop so far: they often continue to fail. So we cannot use methods such as reprimands and punishments on our patients. What works is to give praise when the patient succeeds.

REFERENCE

van Duijvenvoorde, A.C.K., Zanolie, K., Rombouts, S.A.R.B., Raijmakers, M.E.J. and Crone, E.A. (2008) 'Evaluating the negative or valuing the positive? Neural mechanisms supporting feedback-based learning across development.' *The Journal of Neuroscience 28*, 38, 9495–9503.

6

You Need Self-control to Be Able to Cooperate

JAMIE

Jamie is unsure whether he is meant to meet the occupational therapist this afternoon and has asked a healthcare assistant, Marjorie, to check for him. Marjorie has promised to get back to him. Now 2 hours have passed, and Jamie is getting more and more stressed. He goes to the staffroom to ask again, but the door is locked because of a meeting. He knocks. A healthcare assistant, Sebastian, opens the door and says that they don't have time to talk with him since they are in a meeting. He closes and locks the door.

Jamie knocks again. He didn't have time to say that he wanted to talk to Marjorie. Sebastian opens the door again and asks him to stop knocking. They are in a meeting and he'll have to wait.

Jamie kicks at the door. Sebastian opens it again and says sharply: 'You have to wait! We are in a meeting, and the more you disturb the meeting, the longer it will take. Go to your room.' Jamie throws his phone at Sebastian. Then he goes to his room.

Later in the day Sebastian and Jamie discuss the situation. Jamie says: 'I'm sorry, but I was just so angry.'

Sebastian answers: 'You did it on purpose. You just can't do so. But you decided to throw your phone at me. You always have a choice.'

PEOPLE IN AFFECT

The principle 'You need self-control to be able to cooperate' is simple. We often think that we can tell people who are stressed and excited to calm down. But of course people don't usually work that way. A person in affect is a person who can't think normally and who reacts to impulses to a higher degree than usual. Neither will raising one's voice in such a situation have the desired effect.

If we look at the situation in the light of the earlier principles, then we can see that Jamie is unable to control his anger. He does what is most meaningful in the situation from his distressed perspective: he throws the phone at Sebastian. Demands that are too high are being placed on his ability to wait and his ability to regulate his affect. Jamie can't just 'calm down' – his adrenaline level is too high.

THE AFFECT-REGULATION MODEL

We have to handle patients' anger and lack of self-control in many situations – sometimes by intervening immediately to save another patient, and sometimes by just waiting and keeping in the background. What is important, however, is to understand what is happening in situations of behaviour that challenges – and to know how to act in the various phases of the situation. In 1983, Stephen Kaplan and Eugenie Wheeler made a basic model of an outburst of affect (Kaplan and Wheeler 1983), which has since been presented in countless variations. Figure 6.1 shows my version of it (Elvén 2010).

On the *vertical line* of the model we see the intensity of affect, and on the *horizontal line* the time that passes. The *curve* illustrates the progression of affect in a conflict-or-chaos situation. The *horizontal line in the middle* shows how much affect a person can tolerate.

Newborn babies can't tolerate much: they lose control and fail to regulate their affect every time they get hungry. So for them the line is very low. With increasing age, our tolerance of affect improves and the line rises in the model. This we call maturity. As adults we can handle most situations and so the line lies above the curve for most people. For psychiatric patients, however, the line lies considerably lower than for most other people. This means that they lose control of themselves more often than others. This we can call inadequate capacity for the regulation of affect.

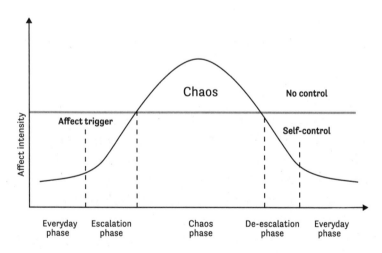

Figure 6.1 The outburst-of-affect model

THE MODEL'S DIFFERENT FIELDS

There are five fields in the model which describe different phases. In the first, the everyday phase, affect intensity is low. The patient is taking it easy or is in a situation that is working well. Then comes a trigger factor: an affect trigger. In Jamie's case, it was that Marjorie didn't get in touch with him. During the escalation phase it is still possible to communicate with the patient. Communication isn't as good as in the everyday phase, but there is still a chance of resolving the situation. In this phase the patient usually still tries to resolve the situation, as Jamie did by looking for the staff. Sometimes the situation moves on into the chaos phase, in which the patient is beyond reach and no longer acts strategically. After a while (because it always passes), the patient gradually calms down and eventually returns to the everyday phase.

The patient's behaviour differs in the different phases and so we too must use different methods if we want to resolve the situation in a good way. (We will discuss this in the coming chapters.)

Most important to take with you from this chapter is that you can only cooperate when you are *under* the line. When the pressure of affect rises over the line, there is no possibility of communicating at all. We get the best cooperation in the everyday phase when the patient has full self-control. In the escalation and de-escalation phases it is more difficult but still possible. But it requires much greater adjustment on the side of the staff to succeed just then. One of the reasons for this is that, in these phases, the patient is fully preoccupied with trying to maintain self-control.

Summary

For patients to be able to cooperate with staff, they must have full self-control. To cooperate is to lend control to someone else. To do this, you must have control. We therefore cannot use methods intended to take control over the patient if we want to increase the level of cooperation.

REFERENCES

Elvén, B.H. (2010) *No Fighting, No Biting, No Screaming: How to Make Behaving Positively Possible for People with Autism and Other Developmental Disabilities.* London: Jessica Kingsley Publishers.

Kaplan, S.G. and Wheeler, E.G. (1983) 'Survival skills for working with potentially violent clients.' *Social Casework* 64, 339–345.

7

We All Do What We Can to Maintain Self-control

FELICIA

Felicia is having a bad day. The morning was tough. She thinks the staff woke her up too early and, since then, things have gone from bad to worse. Felicia couldn't make herself eat breakfast and was bothered the whole time by another patient, Andy, who wanted to talk to her about how bad he feels.

At lunch she discovers that fish is being served. She hates fish and this is the last straw. She leaves the dining room and goes to the washroom. After a while, a healthcare assistant, Cicci, knocks at the door and asks her how she's feeling. 'Like shit,' she says. Cicci fetches the janitor, who unlocks the door. Felicia hits out at Cicci, then squeezes past, runs to her room and sits on the bed.

WHY WE DO EVERYTHING WE CAN TO AVOID LOSING CONTROL

The principle 'We all do what we can to maintain self-control' is simple. We simply do everything we can to avoid losing control. That's not so strange. None of us want to throw furniture around, break windows, scream, fight or bang our head against the wall. So we do what we can to avoid ending up in chaos – especially when we are in the escalation phase (see Figure 6.1).

Effective and good strategies for maintaining self-control are as follows:

- You can try to back off in difficult situations to gain a little calm.

- You can screen yourself off so that you remain in the situation but in such a way that the difficult part doesn't *feel* so difficult.

- You can decide that things will be fine and concentrate on that.

- You can do something familiar in order to feel secure.

- You can seek support from the staff.

Sometimes we use methods that certainly may be effective but may not be as well received by those around us.

Other strategies for retaining self-control are:

- *You can refuse to participate.*
  Just say no. This is perhaps the simplest method – but also the most dangerous. Very many conflicts between staff and a patient begin with a demand to which patient says no.

- *You can tell a lie in order to manage a difficult situation.*
  Research by the Canadian psychologist Victoria Talwar has shown that we lie to protect ourselves if that is the simplest solution. Normal adults, however, usually do this in a sophisticated way, so it is not detected. But quite a lot of patients lie very badly and so we discover

that they are lying right away. Lying requires being good at calculating how other people think, feel and perceive things. Psychiatric patients, regardless of diagnosis, have seldom developed this ability as well as others. We have to take this into account when dealing with a patient we think lies a lot. He is doing his best, but it's not going so well.

- *You can threaten to leave or to hit someone.*

- *You can run away like Felicia (see the case at the start of the chapter).*

- *You can lash out at others so that they keep their distance.*

- *You can seek social affirmation by using bad language.*

The last-mentioned list of methods can be perceived as behaviour that challenges. But it is strategic behaviour – behaviour that is adopted in order to resolve a situation, not to spoil it. This means that, as staff, we must avoid placing a moralistic filter on the behaviour. If you want to change the behaviour, you have to go back to the principles and find out why the behaviour occurred in the first place – so that you can change the conditions and prevent it from happening again. It can be as simple as asking the patient why, in order to then discuss how to find a better solution.

OFFERING A DIFFERENT STRATEGY

The very worst thing we can do is to demand that the patient stop using a particular strategy, without offering an alternative. It is quite effective to talk to the patient about what he can do next time he ends up in a similar situation. But to say 'You mustn't do that. Surely you realise that it will turn out badly' unfortunately doesn't provide enough support for the patient to actually refrain the next time – at least not for most psychiatric patients.

If we look at the affect-regulation model (see Figure 6.1), the implication is that all methods used in the escalation phase must have as their final objective that the patient retains his self-control.

Summary
The patient does his best to maintain self-control. Much of what we think of as behaviour that challenges actually consists of strategies for retaining self-control in order to be able to cooperate. When we counteract the patient's strategies, the result is often a more serious behaviour problem.

8

Affect Is Contagious

CHRISTOPHER

Christopher is a fairly passive guy. Most of the time, he stays in his room at the residence, sitting at the computer. He sleeps a lot.

The ward staff are quite different from him: Ninni is an active person with many interests. She loves talking to the patients about their lives and dreams for the future. Ninni has difficulty with situations in which patients do not engage themselves. If a patient is downright unfriendly, she can get really angry. She has extra difficulty with Christopher because she thinks he's lazy.

Late one afternoon when Christopher is a little tender, he is having difficulty concentrating and sits at the computer just staring into space. The door to the corridor is open. Ninni sees him and asks him to go out to the day room. 'You can't just sit here like a lump all day.' Christopher looks listlessly at her but doesn't react. Ninni gets angry and shouts: 'Christopher! Get up!'

Immediately Christopher gets angry in return: 'Why do I have to go out to the day room? I'm just sitting here. I'm not bothering you, am I? Stupid bitch!' Then he closes the door to the corridor and locks it.

Later Ninni talks about the incident in the staffroom. She thinks Christopher is a good-for-nothing who just lazes about all day long. She's also tired of him shouting and screaming every time someone tells him off. Another healthcare assistant, Nick, who is a very calm person, says: 'Christopher? But that guy is calm – you could hardly find a nicer guy!'

MIRROR NEURON PROCESSES

The principle 'Affect is contagious' was formulated by psychologist Silvan Tomkins as early as the 1960s, but it wasn't until the 1990s that neurophysiologist Giacomo Rizzolatti, in Italy, discovered how it really works: the pattern of activity in a person's brain when he is doing different things is reflected in other people's brains. This means that if someone smiles, then those who see it have the same pattern of activity in their brains as if they themselves had smiled – which can result in them actually doing so!

We humans experience other people's feelings by being infected by them. So it is easier to be happy if one is with happy people, and one is calmed by being together with calm people. It has also been shown that there is some variation in how easily people screen themselves off from other people's feelings. Some people are affected very little by others' feelings, most are affected to some degree by how the people around them are feeling, and others are completely at the mercy of other people's feelings. In psychiatry the last group predominates. Patients are hugely influenced by the affect of the staff and, not least, by each other's affect.

Christopher is sensitive to other people's feelings. Ninni and Christopher are therefore a bad combination. Ninni's enthusiasm and extrovert personality affect Christopher so much that it reduces his ability to manage everyday life. The biggest problem is Ninni's temperament. When Ninni gets angry, Christopher reacts strongly. He cannot regulate his affect as well as most people can and is strongly influenced by other people's affect. This means that he is happiest when he has calm people about him, people who are good at regulating their own affect, and he is stressed by Ninni's energy and temperament.

HOW OUR REACTIONS INFECT PATIENTS

If we return to the principles in the first chapters, then we can say that Ninni, through her personality, places too high demands on Christopher's affect-regulating ability. And since she is a member of staff and he is a patient, she has to change her ways, or shield him by allowing him to be on his own more, if she is to take the responsibility for his well-being that she is employed to take.

This becomes all the more important the more conflicts one has with a patient. I often find that the more conflicts you have with a patient, the more decisive you get in tone of voice and body language. You may start to use marked body language. You may demand eye contact. You may move closer to the patient in demand situations. All these actions increase the transmission of affect and thereby the risk of conflict. Unfortunately, they also result in the patient becoming more determined, which increases the risk of conflict.

To reduce the risk of conflict one should:

- *Never demand eye contact.*
  This is a simple domination tool that often results in escalation of a conflict.

- *Never maintain eye contact for more than 3 seconds in a demand or conflict situation.*
  Psychologist Daniel Stern once said that 30 seconds of eye contact ends in either violence or sex. This is probably not true, but it is most often in this kind of situation that we use long eye contact. Eye contact lasting more than 3 seconds creates a powerful transmission of affect in either a positive or a negative direction – but not in a direction we want in psychiatry.

- *Step back in demand situations and potential conflict situations.*
  By going closer to the patient when making demands or setting a boundary, you increase the patient's stress level. If you take a step backwards at the same time as you make a demand, then the stress of the demand is balanced by the reduced affect transmission.

- *Sit down if the patient is uneasy, or lean against a wall.*
  A calm body is just as infectious as a tense one, but with calm. And we want the patient to be calm.

- *Distract instead of confront.*
  By shifting the patient's focus we remove the transmission of affect that takes place between the patient and ourselves in situations where we want to set limits. You distract by getting the patient to think about something else. In the escalation phase of the model described in Chapter 6, distraction is probably the most important active method to use.

- *Don't take hold of the patient with tensed muscles.*
  Muscle tension is as infectious as affect. If you have
  to take hold of a patient, do it calmly and follow the
  patient's movements. To physically limit the patient
  by holding him tightly will in most cases result in
  violent conflict.

WHY THE ONE WHO WINS LOSES

There is a principle here which probably should have a chapter
of its own, but to which we will return in the chapter on
leadership and authority (Chapter 11) – namely, 'The one
who wins loses.' If a healthcare assistant, nurse or doctor
wins a conflict with a patient, this will not increase the
patient's cooperation. Actually, we don't want *anyone* to
lose. This means that no one wins. Instead of ending up in
a relationship of opposition with the patient, we have to get
the patient to go in the same direction as ours. Methods that
are based on dominance have a different goal and therefore
don't belong in modern psychiatry.

Summary
We are affected by other people's feelings. If we
are together with happy people, we become happy.
Psychiatric patients are often more affected than
others. It is therefore important that staff not be
confrontational or angry in the way they express
themselves. So we need to change our body language
in order to reduce the number of conflicts.

9

Conflicts Consist of Solutions *and* Failures Require an Action Plan

WYATT

Wyatt is lying asleep in the ward. He has an appointment with the physiotherapist at 9 a.m. At 8 a.m. a healthcare assistant, Peter, looks in and says 'Time to get up', and turns on the light. Wyatt pulls the blanket up over his head. Peter takes hold of the blanket and pulls it down a little while saying: 'It's time to get up now. You're going to the physiotherapist at 9 a.m. It would be good if you have time to eat something first.' Wyatt pulls the blanket up over his head again.

Peter opens the curtains wide, fully lighting the room. Wyatt gets up, pushes Peter out of the room, closes the curtains, takes his blanket and gets into bed again. After a while, Peter comes in and says: 'You have to get up now. You were the one who wanted to see the physiotherapist. And you're going to be mad at me if you don't get up. You'll say it was my fault for not waking you. I'm not going to accept that. So now you're getting up. I'm not leaving the room until you get up.'

Wyatt gets up and pushes Peter out of the room. After a while, Peter comes back with three other healthcare assistants. They drag Wyatt under strong resistance to an armchair and push him down into it. Peter says: 'Now you're up. And if you push me again, then it's the belt for you.' The healthcare assistants take the bedclothes with them when they leave.

HOW CONFLICTS CONSIST OF SOLUTIONS

The principle 'Conflicts consist of solutions' is simple. If we consider Wyatt's and Peter's behaviours, one action at a time, then we see that the situation develops according to a simple pattern. One person runs into a problem. He solves it in such a way that the solution becomes a problem for the other person, and so it goes on. The situation develops through a pattern of solutions, which continually cause problems for the other party. The level of violence increases with each solution, finally reaching physical conflict.

This type of conflict can only be solved by one of the parties coming up with a solution that is not a problem for the other. And here comes the interesting part: In most of the cases I have encountered in my work, I have been called on to answer the question, 'How can we make the patient find solutions that are not problematic for the staff?'

In psychiatry it is the staff who are the professionals. It is the staff who are responsible for everyday life and for the patient's well-being and development. Instead of thinking that the problem should be solved by the patient, it would be much simpler if the staff could find a solution that isn't a *problem* for the patient.

WHEN THE STAFF THINK THAT THEY HAVE TO WIN

In the situation above, the staff think they have to win. They also think that they can dominate their way through the situation. In their opinion, the patient has to change his behaviour. This attitude deprives the staff of the possibility to influence – they fail, after all. The risk of failing when you use the methods I have described above is very high. So we have to find solutions with lower risk.

A good solution must be based on not creating problems for the patient. Wyatt's solutions didn't have to become problems for Peter. The problem is that Peter thinks he has to win. And that's when things get out of hand – because Wyatt has no intention of losing. Actually, they both lose when either thinks himself the winner. Peter will have difficulty in being who he should be for Wyatt in everyday life after a conflict like this.

WHY FAILURES REQUIRE AN ACTION PLAN

In the conflict that played out in the example above, we need to apply an effective principle – namely, 'Failures require an action plan.' The principle was formulated in the aftermath of the death of Matthew Goodman. Matthew was a 14-year-old boy with extensive special-education needs. He attended a special school and died from being unable to breathe after having fallen, because his arms and legs were mechanically immobilised with splints and cords.

In the opinion of the court, to use physical restriction of a person's freedom of movement was a failure because it meant that other methods had not succeeded. In this case, the failure led to Matthew's death. Therefore, Matthew's Law was formulated: 'All physical restraints are a pedagogical failure. All pedagogical failures require an action plan.'

If we use the outburst-of-affect model (see Figure 6.1) as we consider Wyatt and Peter's conflict, it is easy to find the trigger factor. It is also very easy to judge whether the methods Peter uses in the escalation phase have the desired effect: that Wyatt can regain his self-control. We can also see that the methods used by the staff in the chaos phase, such as holding him, are not the best imaginable, nor do they improve the situation or the relationship.

AVOIDING PHYSICAL RESTRAINT

Especially in the chaos phase, it is important not to limit freedom of movement. If we carry away or hold a patient tightly, then we will considerably extend the chaos phase. Holding onto a patient with tensed muscles will increase the patient's muscle tension and thereby the stress level, adrenaline flow and risk of violence. It is usually more effective to move away other patients than to move the patient with an outburst of affect. If necessary, one can hold a patient to avoid immediately serious danger to life and health. This can be considered an emergency, and for that reason it would be considered acceptable in most countries.

Using emergency measures is, by definition, something one does in an emergency. Emergencies are rare and unpredictable events. I have occasionally met staff who have told me that they regularly restrain a patient when he acts out. This can never be considered an emergency. If a patient is violent on a regular basis, then it is not unpredictable. Then we must instead identify what demands and expectations we have in the situations where this happens, so that we can avoid them.

In psychiatry it is also permissible in some situations to use mechanical restraint. This must be a doctor's decision, and we must release the patient as soon as things calm down. However, there is no scientific support for mechanical restraint. On the contrary, it prolongs periods of poor psychological health. We see more and more patients with direct flashbacks of mechanical restraint – that is, symptoms of post-traumatic stress disorder caused by psychiatry. This is not in accordance with the mission of psychiatry.

WHY HOLDING OR MECHANICALLY RESTRAINING SOMEONE THREE TIMES IS A METHOD

To mechanically restrain a patient because he threw a chair or something similar is directly unsuitable. Often the patient has already finished throwing things when he is held and mechanically restrained.

Of course, we can use an emergency measure once or twice when a new situation arises. But the third time it happens, it has become a method and not an emergency measure any more. If it happens over and over again, then it is predictable and we must therefore enquire into what has gone wrong. We must modify the situation so that this type of incident doesn't happen again. 'Failures require an action plan.'

Summary
Most conflicts consist of an interplay of solutions: each party in turn tries to solve the problems caused by the other party's solutions. This type of conflict can only be resolved by one of the parties finding a solution that is not a problem for the other party. Unfortunately, we often look for ways to change the patient, when what we should be doing is focusing on not creating new problems for the patient. Because of this, we fail to avoid new conflicts.

10

We Make Demands That Patients Wouldn't Make on Themselves – But in a Way That Works

KELLY

Kelly is tired and doesn't want to shower. She is up and sitting in the day room. But she smells bad. A healthcare assistant, Liz, says: 'What do you say, Kelly? Don't you want to go and have a shower?' Kelly says no. She is not going to shower. Liz says: 'You don't smell so good.' That's none of your business,' answers Kelly.

After a while, Liz offers Kelly a massage. 'But then you'll have to shower first.' Kelly accepts willingly. She loves massage. The shower has become meaningful.

USUAL EVERYDAY DEMANDS

Most of the demands we make in everyday life in psychiatry, and not least in social psychiatry, are about getting patients to do things they wouldn't have done if we hadn't asked them. It can be about getting out of bed, taking a shower and brushing your teeth, but also about calming down, eating politely and not calling other people names.

TAKING AWAY THE PATIENT'S AUTONOMY

Philosopher Martha Nussbaum is of the opinion that all work with people with disabilities to some extent involves taking away their basic right to autonomy. This is an interesting perspective, which may seem somewhat controversial. But I understand exactly what she's thinking. We don't allow patients to decide completely by themselves what they will do and how the day will look – because if they could, they wouldn't be in our care. They are with us because they haven't succeeded in placing relevant demands on themselves.

So we would very much like to decide on the day's programme. We have rules, and we also want to be able to demand certain behaviour of the patients – all for the good of the patient. But that means that we have quite a big responsibility when we work in psychiatry and social psychiatry. After all, we can't just take away all of a patient's autonomy. It is a basic human right to be allowed to decide over your own life. Nussbaum says that since everyone actually has the right to autonomy, then we must have a good argument when we want to limit that right. A very good argument. Every time.

Arguments for taking away patients' autonomy that I think are relevant include:

- *Avoidance of danger*
  The basic principle in most countries is that people may not be locked up as long as there is not a court order giving the right to do so, either by a criminal sentence or through special laws on psychiatric care.

This is the same argument we use in an emergency situation, for example when we grab hold of a person to prevent him from running out into traffic. Therefore, we remove autonomy by custodial care when there is a risk of suicide or serious danger because the person is unable to navigate but wanders around in confusion.

- *Care*
  We use the care argument when, for example, we require good hygiene. When avoiding danger we can have quite far-reaching methods, bordering on or extending into force and compulsion. This is not possible when using the care argument. Taking hold of a person on his way out into traffic would not be seen as excessive, but forcefully brushing a patient's teeth would definitely be crossing the line in many people's opinion. What we can do is to use some pedagogical tricks, and even some manipulative tools, when using the care argument. For example, we can allow ourselves to add swimming to a patient's weekly schedule if we want to ensure that he takes a shower at least once a week; or offer a massage as in the example above. The example of the shower is an interesting case. No one should decide how often I shower; nor should I decide whether a patient should shower. It's part of normal autonomy. But if we think that for social reasons the patient would feel better if he had a shower, then the care argument sets in. But we are not allowed to force the patient.

  Luckily we *are* allowed to motivate. But we must remember the whole time that even this is a restriction of self-determination. It requires a constant ethical reflection over what we want to decide, why and how we then do it.

- *Increasing real autonomy*
  This is the ultimate argument. Many patients cannot handle full autonomy. Normal people probably can't handle it either. Society has followed the implications of this and has limited our autonomy in various situations. A good example is traffic. Parliament has decided that we must drive only on one side of the road. This is an enormous limitation of normal people's right to self-determination. But it means that our ability to travel where we want is greatly increased. If we could drive on whichever side of the road we wanted, then we wouldn't get very far. In school, the curriculum is built on this argument. By deciding what the students should learn in elementary school, we broaden their options for choosing a career. In psychiatry, we use this argument when we limit the activities that a patient can choose, when the patient is unable to form an overview of what is actually possible.

The last-mentioned argument can also be used in situations such as spare time. Some people are good at structuring their time and finding good things to do. They very seldom end up in conflict. Many patients, however, don't have the ability to structure and make good decisions about activities. For some of them, it can be a good idea to structure the time with activities through agreement or suggestion. Some patients need suggestions from which to choose in order to gain autonomy; otherwise, they won't do anything, unless there is something exciting happening that they can't resist. This is not real autonomy, but rather just impulse-governed behaviour. Through limitation of the options, real autonomy can be increased.

OBTAINING A YES

There is a principle that is important to bring up here: 'Make demands so that they work.' I have discovered that, unfortunately, I don't get any fitter by buying running shoes; nor does it help to book time for running in my calendar. If I want to get fitter, I actually have to run. In the same way, it is completely meaningless to make a demand if the patient doesn't act on it.

Sometimes I meet members of staff who say: 'I demand that she get up. Even if she stays in bed for several hours I keep on nagging at her. She's not going to laze around in bed all day long.' For me this is quite absurd. If the patient doesn't get up when we ask, then we have probably made the demand in the wrong way. Instead, we have to find out how to make the demand so that it works and we get the patient to act.

OFFERING STRUCTURES THAT MAKE SENSE

One of the principles we have already considered is: 'People do what makes sense.' This means that if we choose to guide the patient's behaviour in a certain direction (because we have a good argument for doing so), then we can get help from the concept of making sense. There are different ways of doing this. The simplest way is to offer structures and frameworks that prompt the behaviour we want. We discussed this earlier when we considered physical structures, rules and time-related structures for creating predictability. These methods are fundamental for good care. If the rules are good and make sense, if the physical framework automatically leads to good behaviour – and if the everyday routine is predictable – then we have come a long way.

Some activities make no sense to the patients no matter what we do. If these are important activities, then we have to find ways to make them make sense in the situation. This we can do with various methods:

- *Increasing the sense of involvement*
  If patients feel that they have taken part in selecting an activity, then it is easier to get them to participate. This doesn't mean that they need to decide on activities or plan the day on the high, overall level. Sometimes participation in the small things is enough. For example, one might say: 'We were thinking of going for a walk. Where would you like to go?'

- *Creating a sense of belonging*
  If the patient feels noticed by the staff, then his confidence and trust increase. If one has confidence in the staff, then this is often enough to create sense in following directions and living up to demands. It still means that as staff you must ensure that the demands you make are not too high for the patient; if they are, then confidence will wane and behaviour that challenges will increase. One can also try to create a sense of belonging and involvement by letting patients do things together. This requires that at least one patient is able to act as the motor, but the sense of belonging and participation with others can be effective in increasing the behaviour we prefer. We can also get involved ourselves. If we say 'Let's make the bed together', then it is easier to get the patient to participate than if we demand that he do it himself.

- *Preparing patients*
  The better prepared patients are, the fewer conflicts we usually encounter; therefore, it is important to work with plans for the day and the week. One can also make an announcement when there are five minutes left before an activity starts, or to prepare for an ending. The only situation in which this doesn't work well is when we are preparing for an ending in the middle of an activity that has a natural ending at a later time; in this case, time is a blunt instrument that can actually increase the level of conflict. You can't prepare someone to leave a cinema in the middle of a film by saying: 'We're leaving in 10 minutes.'

- *Increasing the sense of sense through outright tricks*
  One example is to use prompts. If we want the patient to get ready to go for a walk, then it helps to hold out his jacket for him. It's simply difficult not to put it on when you hold it out.
  'Done' is another trick. When something has just ended it is easy to start something new. Some activities have a clear 'done', like eating, watching a movie, playing a level in a computer game and so forth. If we prepare for a new activity by saying 'When you've finished watching the movie then we...', then most people will be able to stop and do something else. 'Done' works in group situations too. If we want to start a group activity, then we can serve coffee first. Everyone stops what they are doing in order to drink coffee. And everyone is ready to start when the coffee has been drunk (done).

- *Adding motivational features*
  It could be putting on music when it's time to clean up, making a competition out of a boring task or adding fun to situations where we know there could be chaos – simply making an activity more exciting by adding something interesting or fun.

WHY DISTRACTION IS BETTER THAN SETTING LIMITS

One of the most difficult situations in psychiatry is setting limits. If a patient is engaged in a behaviour that has to be stopped, then the demand is often very clear and corrective in nature. There is unfortunately nothing to show that setting limits leads to changed behaviour in the long run, so at best it is a way of managing a difficult situation – but a risky way.

Norwegian research has shown that violence against staff in psychiatric care begins with limit-setting situations in about 60% of the cases (Bjørkly 1999). Distraction can therefore be a better alternative. If a patient is perceived as disruptive, then he can be reprimanded. But this will not lead to any long-term change; it rather increases the risk that the situation will escalate into conflict. We can increase the sense in not being disruptive by talking about something that interests the patient, capturing his attention, or just getting him to think about something else. A distracting style of work can dramatically reduce the number of conflicts. (We will look more at this in the second part of the book.)

Summary

A part of the job in psychiatry is to make demands on patients that they would not have made on themselves. But it is meaningless to do so if patients don't live up to the demands. We must therefore make relevant demands and do it in a way that means patients can and will succeed in living up to them. Consequently, it is important how the demands are formulated.

REFERENCE

Bjørkly, S. (1999) 'A ten-year prospective study of aggression in a special secure unit for dangerous patients.' *Scandinavian Journal of Psychology 40*, 1, 57–63.

11

You Become a Leader When Someone Follows You

ESTHER

Esther doesn't want to go out on a walk. Anna is trying to get her to come out into the park for a while in the spring sunshine, but Esther refuses. So Anna suggests that they buy an ice cream at the kiosk. Then Esther goes along – she loves chocolate ice cream.

When Anna talks about this later with one of her colleagues, Matt, he says: 'How can you give in to her like that? She should go with you when you tell her. You shouldn't have to bribe her.'

A few days later Esther is sitting in the day room again. Matt comes in and says: 'Time for you to go outside.' Esther says: 'That's not for you to decide.' Matt says: 'You can't sit here and hide. Get out into the sunshine!'

'It's none of your business where I sit, you bloody pig,' Esther answers.

Matt gets angry. But he also knows that he can't force her to go out for a walk then and there. So he says: 'If you don't go out now, you're not getting any lunch.'

HOBBES' GOVERNMENT

The British sixteenth-century philosopher Thomas Hobbes advocated a form of government that nowadays we would call a dictatorship. But Hobbes also claimed that people give up their freedom to a leader in exchange for security, rights and care. If the leader does not manage to satisfy the people's needs in these areas, then they take back their freedom. We have seen many examples of this in recent years, not least in the disintegration of Eastern Europe around 1990 and in the Arab Spring.

In principle, the same perspective applies in psychiatry. Patients give up their right to self-determination in exchange for well-being and security. If we don't succeed on these points, then patients take back their full autonomy, either by questioning or by making a fuss. The patient cannot vote out the staff or the leadership in psychiatry. In that way, psychiatry is a 'dictatorship'.

A few decades ago, one could manage quite well with an authoritarian leadership style as a healthcare assistant, nurse, doctor or psychologist, because patients were used to this style from their childhood. This is no longer the case. Patients are used to being listened to, and many are accustomed to influencing and participating in all kinds of decisions in the family in which they grew up.

One could always discuss whether this development is good or bad, but we still have to relate to the facts. As members of staff in psychiatry today, we need to have a leadership style that lets patients feel involved and listened to if we are to establish and maintain any kind of authority. Unfortunately, staff are not always aware of how badly things go for dictators; otherwise, perhaps we would have made more sure of meeting patients' needs.

HOW YOU GAIN AUTHORITY BY UNDERSTANDING THE NATURE OF POWER

Authority is on the whole an interesting concept. We often fail to create or maintain authority by being authoritarian. Earlier we were looking at the principle 'The one that wins loses'. Matt, in the example above, tried to win but actually lost the conflict. He did not increase his chances of getting Esther out for a walk; nor is Esther likely in the future to feel the confidence needed for her to be able to cooperate with Matt. To create and maintain authority, we must first understand the nature of power.

WHY WE HAVE TO EARN POWER

A psychiatric practice is no democracy. The patients haven't chosen the staff; therefore, the staff have to earn their authority. Just to be clear: there is nothing in the law that requires patients to do what the staff say. The staff, on the other hand, are required to ensure the patients' well-being. So the responsibility for leadership lies entirely on the staff.

This brings us back to the concept of making sense. People do what makes sense in every situation. The staff have to make the desired behaviour make the most sense in each situation – which again brings us back to the tools: the staff must give the patients structures to relate to, both the physical framework as well as rules and activities. The staff have to create trust and a sense of participation in the patients.

FREEDOM OF SPEECH IN SOCIETY AS A WHOLE

One little detail about authority. In democratic countries the authority of parliament and government are tied to freedom of speech. This means that people are allowed to think whatever they want about both parliament and government. They can even say it out loud and write it in the newspaper. If you don't like the government, you are welcome to write an opinion piece or a letter to a newspaper and argue your case; or even just write that that's what you think. You don't really even have to present arguments for your opinions. Let's do a little thought experiment. Someone could write a letter to a newspaper with the following content:

The president is an idiot!

This would be a perfectly legal letter that would not cause any problems whatsoever for the writer. But let us continue the thought experiment. Suppose the next day there was a letter in the paper from the president, saying the following:

In yesterday's paper there was a letter to the editor that described me as an idiot. I don't think it's OK to write such things. The person who wrote it has no knowledge of my abilities. We in power work hard for the people, and I think we deserve more respect.

The president's letter would also be legal. But it would not be received in the same way as the first letter. The reason is that we are actually *allowed* to call the president an idiot. This is something you have to tolerate if you are in power. In this case, as subjects, we are completely under the power of the president. This means that the president has a great responsibility to ensure that the subjects have confidence in the power. The president's imagined letter would not create confidence or authority. On the contrary, it would *undermine* the president's authority, not only in the eyes of the original letter writer but also among those who read the answer.

PATIENTS' FREEDOM OF SPEECH

While in care, patients are subject to the power of the staff in the same way that we all are subject to the power of the government. But patients can't vote out the staff in the same way that we can vote out the government. This entails a special responsibility for maintaining authority and leadership.

The letter above could be compared to Esther's statements at the beginning of the chapter. She ended by calling Matt 'a bloody pig'. Is that OK? That's an interesting question.

Insults are not unusual. They are usually uttered by people with the aim of evening out inequality. If two people have a relationship of equality and one suddenly starts being bossy, then it is not unusual for the other to call the bossy one unpleasant names. He might say: 'Why should you be the one to decide all of a sudden? Blasted idiot!' Then the other person might say: 'Sorry. I shouldn't decide over you. We are equals.' But he could also say: 'What? Blasted idiot yourself!' And then equality is also restored. Two blasted idiots. Is it OK to use insults in this situation? Maybe. So it is OK to use insults towards authority, but it is only *maybe* OK in relationships of equality.

THE RIGHT TO CRITICISE AUTHORITY

So, to answer the question of whether it's OK for Esther to call Matt a pig: yes, actually, it is. Since Matt holds the power, Esther may say practically anything she wants within the framework of the law. The interesting thing is what Matt is allowed to reply. If Matt thinks that their relationship is one of equality, then he will say: 'You mustn't call me bad names. It's not OK.' Then Matt will lose authority, not only

79

in Esther's eyes but also in the eyes of the other patients. And the number of insults will also increase.

If, however, Matt is aware of the power relationship, he will say instead: 'So you might think. But it would be good for you to take a walk in any case. It will do you good.' In this way Matt may be able to save whatever authority there is and it will reduce the number of insults. But threatening Esther with not getting to eat if she doesn't take a walk will not increase his authority.

Sometimes I meet healthcare assistants who have great difficulty in looking at authority in this way. They use arguments such as: 'If Esther is allowed to talk like that, then the other patients will also start doing so. Soon we'll be hearing just anything from the patients.' This is not the case in my experience, however. In reality, most patients are not going to call the staff pigs just because Esther does, in the same way that most of us don't call the people in power bungling idiots just because one person does in a letter to the newspaper. Most patients want to have a good relationship with the staff. The few who don't succeed in this need a greater investment from our side. It is our responsibility to ensure that the patients' confidence and security are so good that the psychological environment does not invite insults to the staff. Then the alliance improves and, with it, health and well-being. And that is our most important task. Matt's behaviour undermines Esther's possibility of managing on her own, and it is therefore badly performed work.

Another objection I have come across is: 'But what if he calls me a whore?' This is much easier, I think. All you have to answer is: 'No, healthcare assistant.' Because it's your occupation that is being questioned, not your person. Because that's how it always is. Insults from a patient are always directed towards the professional, not the person – just as one might think that politicians are idiots in their roles as ministers. Few of us know ministers personally enough to be able to express an opinion of them on the personal level.

LEADERSHIP AND AUTHORITY

There are many other aspects of leadership and authority that could be raised. Most aspects we have covered in earlier chapters, but a little repetition never hurts.

If we want patients to cooperate, we should:

- make sure that what we want patients to do is interesting, understandable and meaningful

- make sure that the physical framework is optimal with regard to space, colour schemes, sound environment and so on

- work actively on creating a good relationship with patients so that we deserve authority.

Create calm by investing in:

- structure and predictability through lists or other plans for what is going to happen

- meaningful rules that the patients follow willingly because they make sense

- being calm ourselves

- not escalating conflicts by adopting a hard line, but rather investing in cooperation

- maintaining authority by not taking it for granted and not misusing it

- avoiding punishment, scolding and reprimands

- making sure that patients feel fairly treated.

Summary

How we get patients to cooperate is unfortunately not something that was included in our education. It has to do with how we handle authority, which is actually something patients hand over to us. We must make it easy for patients to hand over authority to us. This we do best by treating them well and making sure that they feel well and fairly treated.

Part 2

Cases and Action Plans

We begin the second part of the book with a simple metaphor: 'We work in a garage.' When my car breaks down I usually take it to a garage to get it repaired. Basically, I enter into a contract with the mechanic that he will do a job and be paid for it. As a car owner, I expect him to fulfil his part of the contract and he expects me to fulfil my part of the contract. The contract primarily defines who is responsible for what and the expected consequences if one of the parties doesn't live up to his responsibilities. Society has entered into a similar contract with psychiatry: psychiatry is to ensure that patients feel well and, in the long term, can participate in society on the same terms as everyone else.

12

We Work in a Garage

THE MECHANIC'S EXCUSES

Let's assume that I have left my car at the garage because the engine overheats. The mechanic takes a look at it and calls me to say that the water pump is broken and needs to be changed. I am given a fixed price for the work. After a couple of days, I go to the garage to pick up my car. I pay the mechanic. But then the problems begin:

> 'I've done what I could,' the mechanic says, 'but unfortunately the car doesn't work. The engine gets too hot.'

> 'What?' I say. 'But that's what you were meant to fix.'

The mechanic may have some different answers to this:

- 'The car wouldn't cooperate in the repairs. It held on to the bolt so that I couldn't get it loose. I was forced to leave the old water pump in place.'

- 'I told the car to turn down the temperature. After all, the other cars don't get too hot. I think it's a question of motivation. It can if it wants.'

- 'I discovered that the water pump was broken. Things are as they are. I obviously can't do anything about it. At my garage, I look after cars that work. I change the oil and air filters and check that all the lamps work. But cars with defective water pumps can't be my responsibility. So you can take it back. The invoice is for taking care of the car for a couple of days.'

- 'We have had some cutbacks here at the garage. Because of this, I haven't had the time to take care of your car. But it has been here and you must understand that we can't complete all our assignments with the budget we have.'

- 'When I was going to start fixing the car I drove it into the workshop, and while I was doing so, it started throwing engine parts around. They flew all over the place. Obviously I can't work under such conditions. It's a matter of workplace safety. So I pushed it out into the yard and called you. You have to take it home. It's just a nuisance here. But I want to be paid in any case since I didn't have any less work to do. It threw its engine parts about and I had to tidy them up.'

- 'Your water pump is held in by two bolts. They are half-inch bolts. Unfortunately, I don't have any imperial measuring tools. Here at the garage we use metric tools. The reason for this is that research has shown that since most cars are imported nowadays, metric tools are better than imperial measuring tools. Randomly selected cars were repaired using either imperial or metric tools, and metric tools worked on almost all cars, whereas imperial tools worked on only a few. Since our work is evidence based, we threw out all our imperial tools. So I used a 13-mm spanner (a half inch is 12.7 mm), but it slipped and I scraped my knuckles. So now you'll have to wait until the police get here. We have zero tolerance to violence here at the garage.'

We can probably soon agree that I won't be going back to that garage. I expect the mechanic to do his job and take responsibility for service and repairs. I expect him to get help if he can't do the work we have agreed on – just as I expect him to have the necessary tools. Nor do I want to hear any excuses about the garage's finances. And I would never accept that the garage reports my car to the police because the mechanic doesn't have the right tools.

THE CARE STAFF'S EXCUSES

Unfortunately, I have all too often met staff who think like this mechanic. They haven't understood that it is our job to ensure that patients feel well and can manage in life. They also have lots of excuses, ranging from patients' lack of motivation to finances and lack of knowledge. And they make police reports based on zero tolerance that are quite absurd if you consider the mission of psychiatry. Patients are in our care because they can't manage on their own. Our task is to *make sure* they manage.

That patients are condemned to forensic psychiatric care due to violence against staff in forensic psychiatry is our absolutely greatest failing. These patients have most often been sentenced to treatment because they were violent in other situations. The task of forensic psychiatry is to make sure it doesn't happen again. If it still happens when forensic psychiatry has the full responsibility, then we cannot report it to the police; rather, we have to consider what we can do to prevent it from happening again. This can be illustrated by looking at a fairly common situation, as described next.

THE PARKING ATTENDANT

If you get a parking fine, you can look at it in two different ways:

- You can choose to see it as a consequence of having parked in the wrong way.

- You can choose to see it as a consequence of the parking attendant being an idiot.

If you take the first option, there is a good chance that you'll park differently the next day. Then you won't get any more parking fines for a while. This is the better choice.

If you take the second position, then there is a high risk that you'll park the car in the same place the next day. This may lead to another parking ticket. And then the unbelievable happens: you are confirmed in your opinion that the parking attendant *is* an idiot, which doesn't mean that you will park in a better way next time. And every time you get a new ticket, this strengthens your opinion: 'They *are* idiots.'

In the same way, having a zero-tolerance policy against violence means that we don't change our way of working but rather place the responsibility for our professional shortcomings on the patient. When it happens again, we are confirmed in our opinion that the patients are dangerous and violent. Then there is a risk that we will change our methods not in a good direction but possibly in a more violent direction – which increases the risk for violence from the patient – and we get further and further away from fulfilling the task given us by society. It is psychiatry's and social psychiatry's responsibility to ensure that patients feel well.

Summary

This part of the book is about how, in practical terms, we put the responsibility principle into play, find the tools we need for the job and, not least, sort out when we should use the different tools. It is our responsibility to fulfil the assignment given to us by society. And there are no good excuses for failure.

13

Example Situations and Action Plans

A GOOD ACTION PLAN

Before we look more closely at different examples, I will describe how an action plan for a conflict situation could be formulated.

Action plans for conflict situations are simple lists of how one as a member of staff should act when a conflict is developing. The plans should preferably be individual – in other words, relate to a specific patient. Some care staff will immediately say that this is only more unnecessary documentation. But we don't write action plans for situations that have never happened. And for many patients we don't *need* to write action plans, for the simple reason that they are not involved in conflicts that we can't handle.

First you need to make a list of warning signs – in other words, things the patient does when things are starting to go awry. It could be that he talks a lot, has difficulty waiting his turn, raises his voice or bites his nails. I am not talking about things the patient does all the time, but rather about behaviour we have previously noticed just before things went wrong.

There is a reason why I have chosen to have exactly five steps in my action plans. The staff that I have worked with for many years felt their way forward and found that, if you have five steps, you very seldom reach step 5. With more steps or less, you more often get chaotic behaviour.

The five steps of the action plan are as follows:

1. Make room for the patient's own strategies for managing the situation. If this doesn't help, go on to step 2.

2. Here there can be a list of simple ways to distract this specific patient that have worked before. It might be to go to the patient and just be there in order to create calm with one's own calm, to repeat a request in a quiet and calm way, to ask the patient to move on with the programme or to refer to the visual structure. If this doesn't help or if the patient reacts negatively, go on to step 3.

3. Here there can be a list of active distractions that have worked in the past. It may be to talk with the patient about something he likes, joke with the patient or something similar. If this doesn't help, go on to step 4.

4. Here there can be a list of strong distractions. It could be for the patient to run around the hospital area, set aside a current demand in order to work with something the patient is comfortable with and likes, or something similar – the whole time maintaining a calm atmosphere and with a focus on the patient's self-control. If this isn't enough and the patient is approaching or already is in the chaos phase, go on to step 5.

5. Interrupt the situation, possibly by offering a different activity somewhere else or, if the patient is already in

the chaos phase, have other patients leave the room. In rare cases, for example during dangerous behaviour such as a violent fight between two patients, it may be necessary to physically separate the patients with the aid of movement (not holding, which increases conflict and chaos), moving quickly away from the patient afterwards, possibly repeating this several times in close succession, until the patient begins to de-escalate. If this happens often, then training is needed in a scientifically based method. I recommend the Studio III method (McDonnell 2010), a method for physical handling in which there is good evidence of reduced violence, work injuries and patient injuries, as well as improved treatment effect.

It can be an excellent idea to write the action plan together with the patient if you have a good relationship with him. In that case you can also agree on the framework for the plan. For example, I have made an agreement several times with a patient on where he should go when things get difficult. We find a safe place and agree that no staff may approach him when he is there.

Now we will look more closely at different situations and try to understand them in the light of the principles in this book. With help from the affect-regulation model (see Figure 13.1), we will analyse the situations and create relevant action plans.

MARVIN

Marvin is sitting in the day room with a couple of other patients watching TV. In comes a healthcare assistant, Marie, who says: 'Don't you need to go and get dressed, Marvin?' 'Yes,' answers Marvin. Marie starts talking to one of the other patients. After a few minutes, Marie notices that Marvin hasn't got up yet and says: 'Why haven't you got dressed Marvin?' Marvin answers: 'You didn't tell me to.' Marie gets angry: 'Are you going to be cocky now? Time to get going. You must have time to get ready before you go to town.' Marvin answers: 'What? Why are you always mad at me? I haven't done anything. You didn't say that I should get ready right this minute.' Then he throws a magazine on the floor and leaves the room.

Marie follows him and sees him sitting on the bed in his room. After a few minutes, she goes in and says: 'Get dressed now! You have to do what I say. If you don't, I'll see to it that you don't get to go out today. Move it!' Marvin shouts: 'I haven't bloody well done anything! Leave me alone!' He pushes Marie out of the room, and closes and locks the door. Marie takes out her key and opens the door. Marvin slams the door shut. Then he starts throwing his things around and shouting. Marie pushes the alarm.

DEMANDS THAT DON'T WORK

It is not so hard to understand the situation based on the principles we have considered so far. Marie assumes that Marvin understands what she means when she asks him if he isn't going to get dressed. Unfortunately, Marvin *doesn't* understand. Marie's question is really an order. He thinks it is a question. It is not unusual for patients to take things literally and not to understand what we are saying between the lines. The reason for this is that many patients have difficulty in understanding cause and effect in complex situations. This is also the reason why Marvin doesn't understand why Marie suddenly gets angry and asks her why she's always mad at him.

Marvin answers quite correctly that Marie hasn't asked him to get dressed right now – because she hasn't. She hasn't made the demand in a way that works.

Marie immediately assumes that he answers in the way he does because he is being cocky and wants to annoy her. This is why she acts the way she does. She hasn't understood that Marvin is behaving as well as he can. Actually, Marie's affect curve is on the way up before Marvin's curve. Her anger becomes an affect trigger for Marvin. He doesn't understand the situation and his frustration rises. He goes into the escalation phase.

Marie then increases the affect in the situation by going into a mutual affect escalation with Marvin. When Marvin then does what he can to manage the situation, locking himself in to calm down, she confronts him again and raises the conflict to yet another level, so that Marvin loses control. She forgets that Marvin cannot cooperate if he has lost his self-control. Marvin, on the other hand, does what he can to resolve the situation based on the resources available to him.

WHEN TRUST IS GONE AND EVERYONE LOSES

Marie doesn't win. She *tries* to win, but since Marvin locks himself in, she figures that she has not won. So she continues the conflict by raising the alarm. Who loses? They both do. Marie can't live up to her responsibility – to make Marvin feel well – and Marvin doesn't feel well. Who is responsible for this? Unfortunately, we have to say that Marie is. Even if Marvin eventually calms down and is back in the day room the next day, this has been a traumatic experience for him. This reduces the chances that he will develop quickly and well. He can't be expected to have the confidence in Marie that is a prerequisite for him to be able to benefit from his care. Marvin doesn't learn anything from failure.

WHY SITUATIONS ARISE

Situations such as this do arise. Staff misunderstand. Staff sometimes have too high expectations of patients' abilities. Staff act impulsively and primitively instead of thinking things through. I have not been in a single working place where this kind of situation does not occur. What is important is that we, on our side, are able to understand the situation and make sure that it doesn't happen again.

Part of the reason is that Marie was working alone, and that the power structure implies that her version carries the greatest weight. If Marie is like most people, then she will have a hard time admitting that she did anything wrong. She will probably have a tendency to defend her actions in the situation. After all, she has, just like Marvin, only made use of solutions. The problem is that she has a significantly greater responsibility than Marvin does in the situation and ought to have found solutions that didn't cause problems for Marvin.

WHY WE MUST ENSURE THAT IT DOESN'T HAPPEN AGAIN

If we are to have a chance to become better, then there must be contexts where this type of situation can be discussed without Marie feeling guilt or shame. I have seen various ways of doing this. The best method in my opinion is the following: after every conflict between staff and the patient that has involved insults and blows, or the patient locking himself in, throwing things or furniture around, or being mechanically restrained, the work team should sit down and go through the situation using the affect-regulation model as given below (also see Figure 13.1).

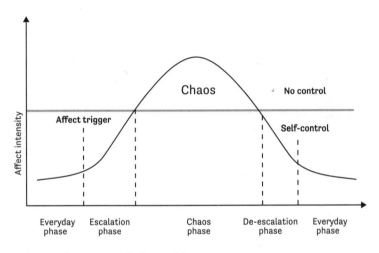

Figure 13.1 The outburst-of-affect model

The everyday phase

In the everyday phase, one asks the following questions:

1. Who said what?

2. What did the staff expect the patient to be able to do?

3. Was the patient actually able to do this?

4. Were there adequate structures available to help the patient do what was expected of him?

The next questions are:

1. Was the staff's behaviour the trigger for the patient's outburst of affect?

2. How can we ensure it doesn't happen again?

3. Should the structures around the patient be changed?

The escalation phase

In the escalation phase (where the greater part of Marvin and Marie's conflict took place) we ask ourselves these questions:

1. Which solutions did the patient try?

2. Were his strategies OK?

3. Was he given the opportunity to collect himself and retain control?

4. Did the staff use solutions that became problems for the patient for which he, in turn, then had to find solutions?

5. Did the staff increase the demands during the escalation phase?

6. Did the staff use any strategies to help the patient retain self-control during the escalation phase (such as creating distance, avoiding eye contact, turning to the side)?

7. Did the staff use body language and a tone of voice that instead reduced the patient's ability to maintain control (marked and insistent body language, direct and demanding eye contact, moving closer or raising one's voice)?

8. Did the staff use any distraction strategies to actively help the patient retain his self-control?

The chaos phase

In the chaos phase, which was brief in this situation, we ask the following questions:

1. Was it a dangerous situation?

2. If it *was* a dangerous situation, was it interrupted quickly and effectively without increasing the level of conflict?

3. If it was not a dangerous situation:

    i. Were the staff able to refrain from intervening?

    ii. Were strategies used with the intention of not increasing the chaos (no eye contact, distance and so forth)?

The de-escalation phase

In the de-escalation phase, we ask the following questions:

1. Was the patient given the necessary space and the peace and quiet needed so that he could land in a good way?

2. Did the staff do anything that caused the situation to re-escalate (such as regulating behaviour, attempting to discipline, pointing out the negative consequences of the behaviour or making new demands before the patient was ready)?

And then we are back to the everyday phase, where we ask the following questions:

1. Which structures must be changed so that this doesn't happen again?

   i. Physical structures?

   ii. Rule structures?

   iii. Time-related structures?

2. Do we have an action plan that we think will work if the same situation arises again?

PROFESSIONALISATION: MOVING THE FOCUS FROM PERSON TO METHOD

These are not very difficult questions in relation to Marvin and Marie's conflict. Marie didn't do very much right as we go through the questions. But since these questions are intended to help us figure out how to avoid a similar situation in the future, the work team's conversation doesn't need to be about what Marie did wrong – but rather about what she can do the next time.

We call this a professionalisation process: we shift focus from person to method. We are actually not very interested in why Marie did what she did or whether it was wrong and what the consequences should be; what we are interested in is what we can do the next time it happens so that we can get better at our job. This means that we don't talk about who is to blame for what happened, but only about method. Preferably the conversation will result in a change to the everyday structure and an action plan that we all can follow next time we find ourselves in something that could become a conflict situation similar to this one.

The changes that are necessary after this event are fairly straightforward:

- If Marvin doesn't get dressed by himself, we should *ask* him to get dressed. We can even offer to help him do so in a friendly way.

- No sarcasm (which increases the intensity of affect, since sarcasm creates shame).

- Make sure that Marvin has a functioning structure for the day, so that he knows what he is going to do. It's a good idea to make an overly clear written plan, showing each step in turn.

In Marvin's case, an action plan could look like this:

1. Stay calm. When Marvin gets riled up, it is often because he hasn't understood. Perhaps repeat the demand calmly and quietly. If this doesn't help, go on to step 2.

2. Show him the structure for the day. It's a good idea to sit down with Marvin. He likes it when you chat with him quietly about how things are going. Then start over. If this doesn't help or if he reacts negatively, go on to step 3.

3. Say sorry if you've had a difference in opinion. He reacts positively to this. Ask him if he's feeling stressed and would like to be alone for a while. If this doesn't help, go on to step 4.

4. Give him the opportunity to get away, perhaps by saying that he can go and have a rest. He usually reacts positively to this. Maybe offer him a magazine. Keep your tone of voice calm and friendly. If this is not enough and he is approaching or already is in the chaos phase, go on to step 5.

5. Allow him to lock himself in his room; he opens up again after about 10 minutes (and seldom makes trouble in the meantime).

HANNAH AND LIAM

The scene is an enclosed yard in a locked ward. There are four patients outside. The weather is nice. Hannah is strolling back and forth, smoking. Liam, Lane and Trey are playing soccer. Liam kicks the ball to Trey, but it goes the wrong way and hits Hannah in the head. Hannah falls down and screams: 'You idiot! You got me right in the head. You stupid dimwit!'

At first Liam doesn't know quite what to say. He's quite keen on Hannah. This didn't go very well. But he also gets irritated. He says: 'I guess you'll have to keep out of the way when we're playing ball. And don't be a bitch about it – it wasn't on purpose.' Hannah replies: 'Don't you call me a bitch! You little shit!'

Liam becomes even more uncertain of the situation. He didn't mean to say bitch – it just kind of flew out of him. He tries to get past her but she stops him by grabbing his sweater. 'And I want you to say sorry, you little shit.' Liam tries to free himself and catches hold of Hannah's hair. She screams loudly and starts kicking him and hitting him with her free hand. Liam hits back and catches her right in the face with his fist.

The staff have noticed the fight and come running. One of them, Casper, takes hold of Liam, who lashes out at him and catches him on the ear. Casper grabs Liam's arms but can't hold him. He gets help from a colleague, Kim, who wrestles Liam to the ground and holds his legs. Hannah keeps kicking and hitting Liam while Karen, another colleague, shouts at her to stop.

Finally, Karen takes hold of Hannah who is still hitting and kicking, now at Karen. Kim releases Liam's legs and takes hold of Hannah. Liam pulls loose and runs off, into the ward. Karen and Casper sit on Hannah, and Karen says: 'Calm down now. We're going to hold you until you calm down.' Meanwhile, Kim fetches the nurse, who gives Hannah a benzo injection. Hannah is now under constant surveillance for the rest of the day and night.

SOLUTIONS THAT ESCALATE THE CONFLICT

A situation like this is dreadful and can have major consequences. It is traumatic for both patients and staff. Patients can be seriously hurt, not least by being held down, and the risk of injury to the staff is also much greater than if they had not taken hold of the patients.

In fact, the risk for everyone involved was significantly increased by the staff's intervention. At the same time it is easy to understand that, as staff, you want to *do* something in a situation like this. You can't just stand there and watch when two patients are fighting. So you try to resolve the situation, and the solutions most often lead to an escalation of the conflict.

WHAT CHANGES ARE NEEDED IN EVERYDAY LIFE?

When I speak with care staff about situations like this one, they always focus on the chaos situation. My thought is always that something is not quite optimal if a situation like this arises at all. So I am keen to talk to the staff about what changes are needed in everyday life. I ask the following questions:

- Was the structure good enough?

- Was there a quiet place to smoke in the yard?

- Was Hannah wandering back and forth because she is unable by herself to create a structure around what she can do in the yard?

- Have we thought about how many patients can be in the yard at the same time?

- Have we considered which activities are suitable for this yard?

- Is the yard's furnishing adequately thought through and divided by function?

WHY WE MUST AVOID VIOLENT SITUATIONS

Staff members often have great difficulty in starting at this end. They want to know how they should have handled the situation when it has already happened. The problem is that it is not enough to have strategies for separating two patients; it is still a dangerous situation that we should do our best to avoid. We should not have situations that are so violent that they require physical intervention. If such situations do happen, then we need to have better methods than holding a patient down. Holding is simply too dangerous.

Simple rules for physical intervention are as follows:

1. Separate the patients by keeping them moving. If you move along with the patient's arm movements, for example, then you can steer them quite easily.

2. Don't use force, but rather movement, for example by reinforcing the person's own movements, which are not directed at the other patient.

3. Go where the patient wants to go – don't resist. Movement is more important than direction.

4. Let go before 10 seconds have elapsed.

The goal is physical distraction, not limitation of freedom of movement. Because that is incredibly dangerous for the patient and often leads to work injuries for the staff. It is therefore my decided opinion that all psychiatric practices should have a 'no-holding goal'. This applies also to forensic psychiatry. Nowadays we have both treatment homes and psychiatric wards that neither hold nor mechanically restrain patients, and we also have forensic psychiatric wards that have taken away the option of physical intervention, including mechanical restraint. Physical interventions are simply unnecessary and dangerous and should not occur.

A GOOD METHOD FOR HELPING THE PATIENT TO SETTLE DOWN

A good way of helping a patient can be to create the possibility for him to withdraw and be alone for a while, if he so wishes, or to offer a group activity that the patient enjoys. We don't need to worry about increasing the risk of fighting by using relation-building efforts that feel good; there are all too many negative experiences associated with the fight itself. Patients don't really want to fight; they want to behave themselves. But fighting was probably the most logical thing to do in the situation.

WHY THE MOST IMPORTANT THING IS TO PREVENT CONFLICTS

The most important thing is therefore what preventative measures could have been taken, both in the everyday phase and in the escalation phase. Were the staff close enough and sufficiently alert? Could they have defused the situation if they had been a little closer? Which distraction tactics would have been effective? If the staff start working with distractions, they usually soon discover that it requires effort. But then we can take control over everyday life, create structure and meaningfulness, divide up the communal spaces into areas for different activities, and so on.

When reviewing the situation using the affect-regulation model (see Figure 13.1), we immediately see that it is primarily in the everyday phase that changes should be made.

Changes in everyday routines could include:

- creating a ball-game area that is separate from the rest of the yard

- creating a quiet and secluded space for smoking

- assessing whether there are generally sufficient staff in the yard

- structuring the work of the staff in the yard; being on watch occurs seldom enough, and active care work could include participating in activities with the patients who most need it, including Hannah.

It is irrelevant to write individual action plans for Liam and Hannah after the event described above. Their behaviour is fully understandable in the circumstances, and so the responsibility falls on the conditions that allowed it to occur. On the other hand, it might be a good idea to write a general action plan for the staff relating to conflicts between patients in the yard or in the day room.

An action plan for conflicts between patients in communal areas could read as follows:

1. Move closer to the situation before it escalates too much, but keep a few metres away. Often it is enough

for a member of staff to be nearby for the situation to calm down. If this doesn't help, move on to step 2.

2. Ask the patients to calm down. If this doesn't help, move on to step 3.

3. Give active suggestions for what the patients can do instead. This could be an activity that is already in progress (card games and the like) or something you know the patients enjoy, such as drinking a cup of coffee. The staff may offer to join in. Bring out something to eat or something else that is a strong distraction. Maintain a calm, friendly tone and focus on the patient's self-control. If this doesn't help, move on to step 4.

4. End the situation by going between the patients, even if they are actively fighting. Get other patients away in order to reduce the pressure of affect. If this isn't enough and the patients are nearing or already in the chaos phase, move on to step 5.

5. In extreme emergencies only, use physical diversion to separate the patients. It must consist of brief interventions where you move with the patient for 5 to 7 seconds and then let go. There must be several members of staff present and the intervention must not have a character of domination or violation. If a situation reaches this stage, then it should be brought up and the staff's response evaluated in the work team.

ELSA

Elsa is always searching out the staff. She asks them what she should do, what time it is, whether the doctor has time to talk to her tomorrow, what's for supper, and lots of other things. She asks the staff whether they have children, whether they have a partner, where they live and if they keep pets. She would probably like to sit in the staffroom and chat all day long.

The staff try to avoid answering personal questions, but sometimes they forget and let slip that they have a cat, or children. Then Elsa has to ask them every day, at the moment they arrive on their shift, how the cat or the children are doing.

In training sessions, the staff have been told not to reply: by having her questions ignored, Elsa will learn to stop asking them. But it is not so easy not to answer. And so the staff have started to avoid Elsa. They stay in the staffroom and nurses' office longer than usual, walk quickly in the corridor and avoid being in the communal areas.

So Elsa has started knocking on the door to the staffroom and the nurses' office several times an hour with little errands: 'Lisa is sad. Will someone come and talk to her?' 'Henry is cold. Can I close the window?' She also continues asking the same questions about food and times that she has always asked. She has also started teasing the staff. She calls Eva 'fatso' and Alan 'dummy' every time she runs into them.

One day, Nasra, a nurse, is walking through the ward. Suddenly Elsa leaps out from behind a door and frightens her so much that she screams and jumps high. Elsa laughs and says: 'Got you there, bloody Arab.'

SOCIAL NEEDS

Elsa is a social kind of person. She loves social interaction. She's just not very good at it. So she does what she can to make contact with the staff. She asks questions, chats and finally scares them.

The staff find her annoying. After scaring Nasra, they also think she's a tease and unpleasant. The word 'tease' is interesting. There are different ways to tease; it can be to bully or to flirt. We see these two variations of teasing very differently from a moral perspective. It's OK to tease as part of flirting if it can be kept at a level where both parties think it's fun. But bullying is never OK. Elsa isn't able to keep it at an OK level. She can't read the nuances that she needs for normal teasing. You have to be able to adjust your teasing depending on how the other person takes it. That's why the staff feel that she is teasing in a bullying way. This, of course, is a problem. They describe her behaviour as intention driven: Elsa *wants* to be irritating.

Actually, what Elsa wants is good contact. She wants to get to know the staff. Some people are introverts; others are extroverts and need contact with other people in order to feel that they exist. You could say that we have different levels of need for other people. Most of us need contact with other people, but we can also be by ourselves. A few prefer to be by themselves. And a few others have such great social needs that they cannot stand to be alone. Elsa most likely belongs in the last-mentioned group.

The problem is that Elsa's level of social competence is fairly low. She is a person with great social needs and low social competence. This is a bad combination. Not many people have this particular combination, but those who do take up a lot of space. Unfortunately, they are often reprimanded more than others are. There is also another factor: the staff have a tendency to try to avoid them. They are very draining to be with, so we work with our backs somewhat turned towards them. Unfortunately, great social need and staff who work with their backs turned is a really bad combination.

Sometimes I hear supervisors and other people say that you should just ignore the behaviour, in order to quench it. This is not a good method. To be ignored is not to be seen, validated, treated with respect and acceptance, supported, included and all the other key words that we use in modern person-centred care. Nor is it effective. Often the behaviour increases if we ignore it, especially when the behaviour we are ignoring is aimed at getting social contact. The social need is not diminished by remaining unfulfilled. So Elsa should not be ignored. Her staff should not work with their backs turned to her. She needs staff who prioritise contact with her.

There are some tricks that can make working with people who have great social needs function well:

- *Fill the need.*
  This is best accomplished by devoting time to the person several times a day. During that time, focus should be on good emotional contact, for example with humour, interesting topics of conversation or by all means exercising together. Half an hour, a couple of times a day, is time well spent; it takes a lot less time if we take the initiative than if we let Elsa do so.

- *Take social initiatives before the person does.*
  Elsa's social initiatives are of rather poor quality. We, who have much better social competence, can take much better social initiatives. We just have to remember

to get there before Elsa does. That is why we cannot work with our backs turned to her and stay in the staffroom or nurses' office.

- *Improve the quality of the interaction.*
  In the situations described above, it is Elsa who acts first. Her initiative comes first, then our reaction – then her initiative, then our reaction. And so it goes on. We can take control of the situation and improve its quality; thereby we also fill the need a little better. We can do this by carrying on the conversation, for example, instead of just answering. When Elsa says 'What are we going to eat?' we could easily ask her what she would *like* to eat. Then we can steer the quality of the interaction and obtain a good and enriching conversation. This improves both Elsa's quality of life and our own.

- *Decide who among the staff should be the one to focus on the patient.*
  One of the mechanisms that is activated when we work with our back to the patient is that we often wait a while before answering or reacting, in the hope that a colleague will handle the situation. So, not only do we have our back to the patient, but we do so for longer than we normally would. This means that the situation often goes on for a little longer than it otherwise would. By dividing up the shift so that we take turns being the primary contact for Elsa, we can treat her in a better way. Additionally, those who are not the primary contact don't need to focus on her at all, so they can get on with their work in peace and quiet.

- *Use as much time as you need.*
  If we try to minimise the time it takes to work with a person with great social needs, then it most often takes more time.

REFERENCE

McDonnell, A. (2010) *Managing Aggressive Behaviour in Care Settings*. London: Wiley.

14

The Principle of the Gentle Approach

FREYA

Freya is stressed. She knows that she may be discharged during the day, but she doesn't feel *ready* to be discharged. When Freya is stressed she gets noisy and disturbs the other patients. She wanders back and forth, grumpy and irritable. The staff know this, and they also know that she doesn't need to be in the ward any longer. She is so well that even the stress of being discharged isn't causing any psychotic symptoms.

Liv, a healthcare assistant, wants Freya to calm down. But she knows that Freya will refuse to do anything she is asked. She cannot be distracted because she will see through the attempt at distraction and refuse. She is certainly not going to let herself be manipulated.

Liv goes up to Freya in the day room and says: 'I know that you are stressed. Actually, I would like to tell you to go to your room or offer you a cup of tea so that you can calm down. But I know that you wouldn't want to do anything I told you to do. Do you have any idea of how we can help you feel a little better?'

We want to round off the book with a final, brief reflection about our approach to people. The book has been about how our behaviour towards a patient is affected by our perceptions about the patient. But we have also described methods both for making demands and handling conflicts. This final chapter will add a simple little truth: it doesn't have to be so complicated. Sometimes it is all about the tone of voice or the approach. It can be as simple as Liv makes it in the case above.

At times I have met staff who think they are working with a low-arousal approach. They have tried distraction ('I told him to drink tea, but if he doesn't want to, there's nothing I can do'). They have tried to adapt their behaviour to suit the situation; they have calmly told the patient to calm down. Actually, what they are doing is trying to adopt the low-arousal approach without changing the basic power relationship between staff and the patient – because underneath it all, they think the patient should understand that it is the staff who decide.

In recent years I have worked to some extent in dementia care. Here the point of departure is completely different. People with dementia have decided over themselves their whole lives. Now that things have become sufficiently difficult, they are moved into a context where suddenly there are *staff* who are meant to decide over them. But at the same time they have so much difficulty in understanding and remembering where they are and why, that they don't understand that they need help in managing their everyday lives. This means that they most often refuse to take orders from the staff. The staff still have to make the necessary demands, but in such a way that the person feels that he himself is the one choosing what must be done.

If we extrapolate this to psychiatry, then everything gets so much simpler. Actually, we are back to the concept of involvement, which we discussed earlier. In the above case, if Freya feels that Liv takes her seriously and meets her in her situation, then maybe she will be able to find a way out of her stress. Liv asks for cooperation, but she does it by validating Freya's perception of things. Freya is stressed. Liv acknowledges this. Freya needs to know that it's OK to be stressed – but also that Liv knows that it's a difficult situation and would like to offer a way out. This is one of many ways to work with the gentle approach.

JOEL

Joel should go to bed. He knows it. It's nearly midnight and he needs his sleep in order to feel well. He paces back and forth in the corridor and waits for someone from the staff to tell him to go to bed – except that he doesn't think the staff have the right to decide when he should go to bed. He's building up anger against the staff because they think they can decide such things.

Tony, a healthcare assistant, walks by with another patient, Janet. He says to Joel: 'Janet's bed needs attention and I'm on my way to fix it. It squeaks every time she moves, so I'm going to oil it. Do you want to help? And shall we take a look at yours afterwards, so you can go to bed?'

THE FINE DETAIL

Another way of working with the gentle approach is the subclause. In the example above, Tony focuses not on the demand but on something else that gives Joel a chance to go to bed without actually submitting to the staff's authority. Putting the demand in the subclause takes away Joel's sense of subordination. At the same time Tony offers involvement in the form of the question and in the form of belonging in the situation where they fix the bed – but all in a gentle approach.

Staff often want to be direct and clear. That's fine, except that sometimes patients have trouble with confrontation. To work with low arousal is not just saying the same things but without raising your voice; it's about adjusting your work so that the patient's affect does not rise. This can be done through good planning and the methods we have discussed in this book. But it's possible to take it one step further with the gentle approach.

It's not about spoiling the patient or being namby-pamby. It's about planning and carrying out the work in a way that is effective and gives the patient a sense of acting for himself. It's not the work itself that we do differently; it's just a small way of further increasing the patient's possibility of succeeding. A little pedagogical fine detail.

CLARITY AND INVOLVEMENT BELONG TOGETHER

The most important thing is to keep your eye on the goal. Tony's goal is for Joel to go to bed. Liv's goal is for Freya to calm down. Neither Tony nor Liv pander to the patient. They are actually quite clear about what they want the patients to do, but as mentioned, they have a gentle way of making contact with them.

The opposite is pussyfooting staff. Sometimes I come across staff who find patients' emotional outbursts so difficult that they try to avoid the patient getting anxious or angry. As a result, they don't dare make demands and are much too soft in their approach, and also unclear about the goal. This is devastating. If the staff pussyfoot, then the patient sees them as incompetent. Pussyfooting staff don't pussyfoot because they want to shield the patient from getting anxious or angry; they pussyfoot to avoid the anxiety they themselves feel when the patient gets anxious or angry. This is not what Liv and Tony are doing. They are implementing a planned pedagogical approach with a clear objective, but with the help of good pedagogical tools such as validation, involvement and subclauses. And in this way the gentle approach becomes an excellent way to help the patient accomplish what he needs to do – at the same time as he has a good day and feels both seen and respected.

Exactly what the assignment is.

Part 3

Extra Material

Study Materials

I am glad that you are interested in going into more depth. Here are some questions you can use when talking about the book, principle by principle. You could potentially spend 15 to 30 minutes on this at staff meetings and gradually work your way through the book.

PART 1: PRINCIPLES

Chapter 1: Always Identify Who It Is That Has a Problem

Much of what we perceive to be behaviour that challenges is only a problem to *us*. Often the patient sees it as a solution.

Discuss

- Think of examples of situations where something that you thought of as problematic behaviour definitely wasn't a problem for the patient.

- Was it clear in any of these situations that the difference in how staff and the patient saw the situation led to an escalation of the conflict?

Chapter 2: People Behave Well If They Can

This principle is one of many possible formulations of Ross W. Greene's statement: 'Kids do well if they can.' I think it is the formulation with the most power.

Here is a list of abilities on which, in my opinion, we often place too high demands:

- the ability to calculate cause and effect in complex situations

- the ability to structure and carry out activities

- the ability to remember while thinking

- the ability to restrain impulses

- endurance

- flexibility

- social skills

- sensitivity to stress

- the ability to say yes

- the ability to calm down and stay calm.

Discuss

- On which abilities have you had too high expectations? Think of a few situations for each ability.

- Think of situations where things have gone badly, and where you can identify where your expectations were too high. How can you avoid similar situations in the future and adjust so that patients can live up to expectations?

- Is it enough to focus on changing our expectations or is it the way we think about patients that needs changing?

Chapter 3: People Do What Makes Sense
Discuss

- Think of situations where, when you think it through, you can fully understand why the patient acted as he did.

- Think of situations in your own life where the way you acted perhaps wasn't how those around you wanted, but you did it anyway because it was what made the most sense at the time. Was your behaviour in those situations the best after all, in the long-term perspective?

Chapter 4: The One Who Takes Responsibility Can Make a Difference
Discuss

- Think of situations where you, as staff, try to pass on responsibility.

- Are there some patients who are always described with words such as 'stubborn'?

- Are there patients who you try to send on to secure facilities?

Chapter 5: Those Who Are Used to Failing Learn Nothing from Failing One More Time
Discuss

- Think of situations that you handled based on the assumption that the patient learns from failure.

- What consequences does this assumption have for your daily work and for the patients?

Chapter 6: You Need Self-control to Be Able to Cooperate

This principle is best discussed together with the next one.

Chapter 7: We All Do What We Can to Maintain Self-control

Discuss

- Think of situations where what you thought of as behaviour that challenges was actually the patient's strategy for retaining self-control.

- How will this insight affect your work from now on?

Chapter 8: Affect Is Contagious

Discuss

- Think of situations where your affect is transmitted to the patients. It could be anger or uneasiness (stress), but also joy and enthusiasm.

- See if you can think of situations where the patients' affect infected you to the point where you lost your overview and your ability to hold the situation together.

- Can you think of potential strategies for minimising the risk of this happening?

Chapter 9: Conflicts Consist of Solutions *and* Failures Require an Action Plan
Discuss

- Think of situations where conflicts between you and patients have had the structure described by this principle.

- Think of situations where conflicts between patients have followed this pattern. How could you have intervened in these situations? It's a good idea to think in concrete terms based on the situations you have come up with.

Chapter 10: We Make Demands That Patients Wouldn't Make on Themselves – But in a Way That Works
Discuss

- Which methods do you use in your daily work to get patients to say yes? Use the list beginning on page 72 of this book as starting point, but also try to come up with methods of your own that I haven't considered.

- Which distractions do you use? It's a good idea to talk about a specific patient and write down the distractions each of you uses, so that you can share them.

Chapter 11: You Become a Leader When Someone Follows You
This chapter is about authority.
Discuss

- What do you do to get patients to give you authority? Try to give examples of concrete strategies.

PART 2: CASES AND ACTION PLANS

Chapter 12: We Work in a Garage

Now that you have come this far, it might be a good idea to go back to the responsibility principle.

Discuss

- How well does the garage metaphor fit your work? Do you work in a garage or do you have a tendency to:
  - ▸ lay the blame for the patient's lack of success on his unwillingness to cooperate?
  - ▸ feel that the patient is not doing his best in the situation?
  - ▸ use methods that you are comfortable with even when you have been advised that the patient needs other methods?

Chapter 13: Example Situations and Action Plans

For this chapter you will find materials for discussion in the scenarios and action plans included in the main text.

Chapter 14: The Principle of the Gentle Approach

Discuss

- Think of situations where you have succeeded specifically because you used the gentle approach:
  - ▸ with the question about cooperation, as in Freya's case
  - ▸ with the subclause, as in Joel's case.
- Think of other ways in which you use the gentle approach.

Further Reading

It makes me glad that you are reading this book and are interested in going into more depth in the knowledge on which it is based. Here I present the background to the ideas and methods included in the book, going in order from first page to last. This means that I will repeat myself along the way, but also that the context of the principles will become more clear.

PART 1: PRINCIPLES

Chapter 1: Always Identify Who It Is That Has a Problem

The thoughts in this chapter were formulated by Andrew McDonnell in the book:

> McDonnell, A. (2010) *Managing Aggressive Behaviour in Care Settings*. London: Wiley.

They also form the basis for the book:

> Elvén, B.H. (2010) *No Fighting, No Biting, No Screaming: How to Make Behaving Positively Possible for People with*

Autism and Other Developmental Disabilities. London: Jessica Kingsley Publishers.

Chapter 2: People Behave Well If They Can

The expression 'People behave well if they can' is one of many possible formulations of Ross W. Greene's statement: 'Kids do well if they can.' I think it is the formulation that carries the most weight. The statement is taken from the book:

> Greene, R.W. (2014) *The Explosive Child: A New Approach for Understanding and Parenting Easily Frustrated, Chronically Inflexible Children.* New York, NY: Harper Paperbacks.

If you want to read more about executive functions (on which such high demands are placed in Zoe's case), you would benefit from reading the following:

> Gazzaniga, M.S., Ivry, R.B. and Mangun, G.R. (2013) *Cognitive Neuroscience.* New York, NY: W.W. Norton.

Greene himself keeps a continuously updated list of references for relevant research on his website (www.livesinthebalance.org).

List of abilities

The list of abilities on which we often find ourselves placing too high demands (see pages 24–26) is my own, but for each ability there are a host of references:

- *Ability to calculate cause and effect in complex settings*
  A good summary of this concept can be found in:

> Happé, F. (2013) 'Weak Central Coherence.' In F.R. Volkmar (ed.) *Encyclopedia of Autism Spectrum Disorders.* New York, NY: Springer.

- *Ability to structure, plan and carry out activities*

  Gazzaniga, M.S., Ivry, R.B. and Mangun, G.R. (2013) *Cognitive Neuroscience*. New York, NY: W.W. Norton.

- *Ability to remember while thinking*

  Baddeley, A. (2007) *Working Memory, Thought, and Action* (Oxford Psychology Series). Oxford: Oxford University Press.

- *Ability to restrain impulses*

  Gazzaniga, M.S., Ivry, R.B. and Mangun, G.R. (2013) *Cognitive Neuroscience*. New York, NY: W.W. Norton.

- *Ability to endure*
  A good science-journalism article on the subject can be found here:

  Lehrer, J. (2009) 'Don't.' *The New Yorker*, 18 May. Available at www.newyorker.com/reporting/2009/05/18/090518fa_fact_lehrer, accessed on 4 August 2016.

- *Ability to be flexible*
  This is an older definitive article:

  Scott, W.A. (1962) 'Cognitive complexity and cognitive flexibility.' *American Sociological Association 25*, 405–414.

- *Social skills*

  Frith, U. (2003) *Autism: Explaining the Enigma*. London: Wiley.

- *Sensitivity to stress*

  Elvén, B.H. (2010) *No Fighting, No Biting, No Screaming: How to Make Behaving Positively Possible for People with*

Autism and Other Developmental Disabilities. London: Jessica Kingsley Publishers.

- *Ability to say yes*

  DiStefano, C., Morgan, G.B. and Motl, R.W. (2012) 'An examination of personality characteristics related to acquiescence.' *Journal of Applied Measurement 13*, 1, 41–56.

- *Ability to calm down and stay calm*

  Diekhof, E.K., Geier, K., Falkai, P. and Gruber, O. (2011) 'Fear is only as deep as the mind allows: a coordinate-based meta-analysis of neuroimaging studies on the regulation of negative affect.' *Neuroimage 58*, 1, 275–285.

  Sjöwall, D., Roth, L., Lindqvist, S. and Thorell, L.B. (2013) 'Multiple deficits in ADHD: executive dysfunction, delay aversion, reaction time variability, and emotional deficits.' *Journal of Child Psychology and Psychiatry 54*, 6, 619–627.

Chapter 3: People Do What Makes Sense

You can read about understandable physical frameworks in:

Elvén, B.H. (2014) 'Fysiske rammer og problemskabende adfærd.' In Kaas and Skovgaard Schmidt, *Særforanstaltninger – anbefalinger til god praksis for organisering, samarbejde og borgerinddragelse.* Odense: Socialstyrelsen.

Norman, D. (1988) *The Psychology of Everyday Things.* New York, NY: Basic Books.

On structure and predictability as the basis for meaningfulness:

> Kabot, S. and Reeve, C. (2012) *Building Independence: How to Create and Use Structured Work Systems*. Lenexa, KS: Autism Asperger Publishing Co.

Chapter 4: The One Who Takes Responsibility Can Make a Difference

This principle is derived from:

> Weiner, B. (1995) *Judgments of Responsibility: A Foundation for a Theory of Social Conduct*. New York, NY: Guilford Press.

You can read about Dave Dagnan's work in:

> Dagnan, D. and Cairns, M. (2005) 'Staff judgements of responsibility for the behaviour that challenges of adults with intellectual disabilities.' *Journal of Intellectual Disability Research 49*, 1, 95–101.

This chapter includes a discussion of punishment. It needs to be pointed out that the concept of punishment used in this book is the same as that used in the general population. It is thus not the concept of punishment used in behaviourism. Research and theories that support the negative effects of punishment can be found in:

> Gershoff, E.T. (2002) 'Corporal punishment by parents and associated child behaviors and experiences: a meta-analytic and theoretical review.' *Psychological Bulletin 128*, 4, 539–579.

> Shutters, S.T. (2013) 'Collective action and the detrimental side of punishment.' *Evolutionary Psychology 11*, 2, 327–346.

Sigsgaard, E. (2005) *Scolding: Why It Hurts More Than It Helps*. New York, NY: Teachers College Press.

On legitimising effects:

Gneezy, U. and Rustichini, A. (2000) 'A fine is a price.' *The Journal of Legal Studies 29*, 1, 1–17.

On differing tendencies to punish:

de Quervain, D.J.F., Fischbacher, U., Treyer, V., Schellhammer, M. *et al.* (2004) 'The neural basis of altruistic punishment.' *Science 305*, 1254–1258.

On why we punish:

Boyd, R., Gintis, H., Bowles, S. and Richerson, P.J. (2003) 'The evolution of altruistic punishment.' *Proceedings of the National Academy of Science USA 100*, 6, 3531–3535.

Chapter 5: Those Who Are Used to Failing Learn Nothing from Failing One More Time

The chapter builds on the following article:

van Duijvenvoorde, A.C.K., Zanolie, K., Rombouts, S.A.R.B., Raijmakers, M.E.J. and Crone, E.A. (2008) 'Evaluating the negative or valuing the positive? Neural mechanisms supporting feedback-based learning across development.' *The Journal of Neuroscience 28*, 38, 9495–9503.

Chapter 6: You Need Self-control to Be Able to Cooperate

Original article by Kaplan and Wheeler:

Kaplan, S.G. and Wheeler, E.G. (1983) 'Survival skills for working with potentially violent clients.' *Social Casework 64*, 339–345.

The model was first published in:

Elvén, B.H. (2010) *No Fighting, No Biting, No Screaming: How to Make Behaving Positively Possible for People with Autism and Other Developmental Disabilities*. London: Jessica Kingsley Publishers.

It is also possible to go into more depth in:

Diekhof, E.K., Geier, K., Falkai, P. and Gruber, O. (2011) 'Fear is only as deep as the mind allows: a coordinate-based meta-analysis of neuroimaging studies on the regulation of negative affect.' *Neuroimage 1*, 58, 275–285.

Sjöwall, D., Roth, L., Lindqvist, S. and Thorell, L.B. (2013) 'Multiple deficits in ADHD: executive dysfunction, delay aversion, reaction time variability, and emotional deficits.' *Journal of Child Psychology and Psychiatry 54*, 6, 619–627.

Chapter 7: We All Do What We Can to Maintain Self-control

One can go into depth in the way of thinking by reading:

Elvén, B.H. (2010) *No Fighting, No Biting, No Screaming: How to Make Behaving Positively Possible for People with Autism and Other Developmental Disabilities*. London: Jessica Kingsley Publishers.

On the strategy of talking to the patient:

Rollnick, S. and Miller, W.R. (1995) 'What is motivational interviewing?' *Behavioural and Cognitive Psychotherapy* *23*, 325–334.

A good scientific-journalism article on lying:

Bronson, P. (2008) 'Learning to lie.' *New York Magazine*, 8 February. Available at http://nymag.com/news/features/43893, accessed on 4 August 2016.

Chapter 8: Affect Is Contagious

The concept of affect contagion comes from:

Tomkins, S. (1962) *Affect, Imagery, Consciousness* Volume I. London: Tavistock.

Tomkins, S. (1963) *Affect, Imagery, Consciousness* Volume II: *The Negative Affects*. New York, NY: Springer.

Tomkins, S. (1991) *Affect, Imagery, Consciousness* Volume III: *The Negative Affects – Anger and Fear*. New York, NY: Springer.

Scientific basis:

Hatfield, E., Cacioppo, J.T. and Rapson, R.L. (1993) 'Emotional contagion.' *Current Directions in Psychological Science 2*, 3, 96–99.

Mirror neuron research comes from:

Rizzolatti, G. and Craighero, L. (2004) 'The mirror-neuron system.' *Annual Review of Neuroscience 27*, 169–192.

Strategies for reducing the pressure of affect are from the low-arousal approach:

Elvén, B.H. (2010) *No Fighting, No Biting, No Screaming: How to Make Behaving Positively Possible for People with Autism and Other Developmental Disabilities*. London: Jessica Kingsley Publishers.

McDonnell, A. (2010) *Managing Aggressive Behaviour in Care Settings*. London: Wiley.

Chapter 9: Conflicts Consist of Solutions *and* Failures Require an Action Plan

You can read about Matthew Goodman at: www.inclusiondaily.com/news/institutions/nj/bancroft.htm

Physical restraint is extremely dangerous. One study showed that, after physical restraint, 18.8% of staff were injured as well as 17.6% of those they restrained. See:

Legget, J. and Silvester, J. (2003) 'Care staff attributions for violent incidents involving male and female patients.' *British Journal of Clinical Psychology 42*, 393–406.

Scientific documentation on restraint-related deaths can be found here:

Aiken, F., Duxbury, J., Dale, C. and Harbison, I. (2011) *Review of the Medical Theories and Research Relating to Restraint Related Deaths*. Lancaster: Caring Solutions (UK), University of Central Lancashire.

Nunno, M.A., Holden, M.J. and Tollar, A. (2006) 'Learning from tragedy: a survey of child and adolescent restraint fatalities.' *Child Abuse and Neglect 30*, 1333–1342.

Paterson, B., Bradley, P., Stark, C., Saddler, D., Leadbetter, D. and Allen, D. (2003) 'Deaths associated with restraint use in health and social care in the UK: The results of a preliminary survey.' *Journal of Psychiatric and Mental Health Nursing 10*, 3–15.

On how a decrease in restraints decreases injuries:

Holstead, J., Lamond, D., Dalton, J., Horne, A. and Crick, R. (2010) 'Restraint reduction in children's residential facilities: implementation at Damar Services.' *Residential Treatment for Children & Youth 27*, 1–13.

Chapter 10: We Make Demands That Patients Wouldn't Make on Themselves – But in a Way That Works

Martha Nussbaum's thoughts can be found in:

Nussbaum, M.C. (2007) *Frontiers of Justice: Disability, Nationality, Species Membership (The Tanner Lectures on Human Values)*. Boston, MA: Harvard University Press.

On violence against staff who set boundaries:

Bjørkly, S. (1999) 'A ten-year prospective study of aggression in a special secure unit for dangerous patients.' *Scandinavian Journal of Psychology 40*, 1, 57–63.

On distraction:

Elvén, B.H. (2010) *No Fighting, No Biting, No Screaming: How to Make Behaving Positively Possible for People with Autism and Other Developmental Disabilities*. London: Jessica Kingsley Publishers.

McDonnell, A. (2010) *Managing Aggressive Behaviour in Care Settings.* London: Wiley.

Smith, R.E. (1973) 'The use of humor in the counterconditioning of anger responses: a case study.' *Behavior Therapy 4,* 4, 576–580.

Chapter 11: You Become a Leader When Someone Follows You

Hobbes' thoughts on power are taken from:

Hobbes, T. (1651/1982) *Leviathan.* New York, NY: Penguin Classics.

Rawls' thoughts are from:

Rawls, J. (1971) *A Theory of Justice.* Cambridge, MA: Belknap Press of Harvard University Press.

Martha Nussbaum's thoughts on autonomy are from:

Nussbaum, M.C. (2007) *Frontiers of Justice: Disability, Nationality, Species Membership (The Tanner Lectures on Human Values).* Boston, MA: Harvard University Press.

PART 2: CASES AND ACTION PLANS

The garage has zero tolerance for violence. Zero tolerance has been shown to have a negative effect on psychiatric care. If you want to look at this in more depth, you can read:

Middleby-Clements, J.L. and Grenyer, B.F.S. (2007) 'Zero tolerance approach to aggression and its impact upon mental health staff attitudes.' *Australian and New Zealand Journal of Psychiatry 41,* 187–191.

Paterson, B., Miller, G., Leadbetter, D. and Bowie, V. (2008) 'Zero tolerance and violence in services for people with mental health needs.' *Mental Health Practice 11*, 8, 26–31.

The model with the different phases builds on:

Kaplan, S.G. and Wheeler, E.G. (1983) 'Survival skills for working with potentially violent clients.' *Social Casework 64*, 339–345.

Whitaker, P. (2001) *Behaviour that challenges and Autism: Making Sense, Making Progress*. London: National Autistic Society.

The model was used for the first time in:

Bendixen, C., Esbensen, A., Pedersen, L.M., Hansen, L., Hansen, S.G. and Pøhler, L. (2005) *Magtanvendelse i Folkeskolen*. København: Center for ligebehandling af handicappede og Børnerådet i samarbejde med Undervisningsministeriet.

The action plan model comes from:

Björne, P., Andresson, I., Björne, M., Olsson, M. and Pagmert, S. (2012) *Utmanande beteenden, utmanande verksamheter*. Malmö: Stadskontoret.

You can read more on physical interventions and Studio III in:

McDonnell, A. (2010) *Managing Aggressive Behaviour in Care Settings*. London: Wiley; and at www.studio3.org.